Ophthalmology
 **IN** *focus*

For Elsevier

Commissioning Editor: *Ellen Green*
Project Development Manager: *Helen Leng*
Project Manager: *Frances Affleck*
Designer: *George Ajayi*

Ophthalmology

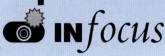

IN *focus*

Jack J Kanski MD MS FRCS FRCOphth

Honorary Consultant Ophthalmic Surgeon
Prince Charles Eye Unit
King Edward VII Hospital
Windsor
UK

Brad Bowling FRCSEd (Ophth), FRCOphth

Specialist Registrar
Oxford Eye Hospital
Oxford
UK

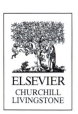

ELSEVIER
CHURCHILL
LIVINGSTONE

EDINBURGH   LONDON   NEW YORK   OXFORD   PHILADELPHIA   ST LOUIS   SYDNEY   TORONTO 2005

ELSEVIER | CHURCHILL
LIVINGSTONE
An imprint of Elsevier Limited

© Longman Group Ltd 1984, 1992
© Pearson Professional Limited 1997
© 2005, Elsevier Limited. All rights reserved.

First published as Colour Aids Ophthalmology 1984
First Colour Guide edition 1992
Second Colour Guide edition 1997
Reprinted 1998, 2001
First in Focus edition 2005
    Reprinted 2006

ISBN 0 443 10030 6

British Library Cataloguing in Publication Data
A catalogue record for this book is available from the British Library

Library of Congress Cataloguing in Publication Data
A catalogue record for this book is available from the Library of Congress

Note
Medical knowledge is constantly changing. Standard safety precautions must be followed, but
as new research and clinical experience broaden our knowledge, changes in treatment and
drug therapy may become necessary or appropriate. Readers are advised to check the most
current product information provided by the manufacturer of each drug to be administered to
verify the recommended dose, the method and duration of administration, and
contraindications. It is the responsibility of the practitioner, relying on experience and
knowledge of the patient, to determine dosages and the best treatment for each individual
patient. Neither the Publisher nor the author assumes any liability for any injury and/or
damage to persons or property arising from this publication.

The Publisher

ELSEVIER   your source for books,
journals and multimedia
in the health sciences

www.elsevierhealth.com

Working together to grow
libraries in developing countries
www.elsevier.com | www.bookaid.org | www.sabre.org

ELSEVIER   BOOK AID
International   Sabre Foundation

The
publisher's
policy is to use
paper manufactured
from sustainable forests

Printed in China

Acknowledgements

We are very grateful to the following colleagues for providing us with illustrations: M Batterbury (Fig. for Question 28); Prof A Bird (Figs 50, 217, 218, 242, 243, 248); R Chopdar (Fig. for Question 101); Eye Academy (Fig. for Question 95); J Federman (Fig. 229); R Marsh (Fig. 62); B Mathalone (Figs 67, 250, 258, 259); C Migdal (Figs 70, 69, 237); A Mitchell (Fig. 56); P Morse (Figs 235, 265); T Rahman (Figs 136, 200); A Ridgeway (Fig. 98); J Shilling (Fig. 132); A Shun-Shin (Figs 44, 48, 125, 232, 245); D Spalton (Fig. 128); V Tanner (Fig. 43); D Taylor (Fig. 167).

Contents

1. Blepharitis   2
2. Non-neoplastic eyelid nodules   4
3. Benign tumours of the eyelids   6
4. Premalignant and malignant tumours of the eyelids   8
5. Ptosis   10
6. Entropion, ectropion and trichiasis   12
7. Thyroid eye disease   14
8. Orbital tumours   16
9. Miscellaneous orbital disease   18
10. Acute conjunctivitis   20
11. Chronic conjunctivitis   22
12. Conjunctival tumours   24
13. Keratoconjunctivitis sicca and cicatrizing conjunctivitis   26
14. Suppurative keratitis   28
15. Herpes simplex infection   30
16. Herpes zoster ophthalmicus   32
17. Corneal dystrophies   34
18. Peripheral corneal ulceration   36
19. Disorders of corneal size and shape   38
20. Episcleritis and scleritis   40
21. Anterior uveitis   42
22. Posterior uveitis – infections   44
23. Non-infectious intermediate and posterior uveitis   46
24. Idiopathic multifocal white dot syndromes   48
25. Primary open-angle glaucoma   50
26. Secondary open-angle glaucomas   52
27. Primary angle-closure glaucoma   54
28. Secondary angle-closure glaucomas   56
29. Developmental glaucomas   58
30. Age-related cataract   60
31. Miscellaneous disorders of the lens   62
32. Diabetic retinopathy   64
33. Retinal vascular occlusion   66
34. Miscellaneous retinopathies   68
35. Age-related macular degeneration   70
36. Acquired maculopathies   72
37. Dystrophies of the fundus   74
38. Retinal detachment   76
39. Tumours of the uvea   78
40. Tumours of the retina and optic nerve head   80
41. Acquired optic nerve disorders   82
42. Congenital optic disc anomalies   84
43. Childhood strabismus (squint)   86
44. Third, fourth and sixth nerve palsies   88
45. Trauma   90

Questions   92

Answers   145

Index   169

1 Blepharitis

Definition	Very common chronic inflammation of the eyelid margins.
Classification	Divided into anterior and posterior forms: the former may be staphylococcal or seborrhoeic; a mixed picture is typical, however.
Aetiology	Causative factors:

- *Staphylococcal*: chronic infection of the bases of the lashes – common in patients with eczema
- *Seborrhoeic*: usually associated with seborrhoeic dermatitis – involves excess lipid production by eyelid glands, converted to fatty acids by bacteria
- *Posterior*: dysfunction of the meibomian glands of the posterior lid margins – common in patients with acne rosacea.

Clinical features

Symptoms: usually worse in the morning, include grittiness, burning and redness, stickiness and crusting of the lids.

Signs

- *Staphylococcal*: dandruff-like scaling, mainly around the eyelash bases (Fig. 1)
- *Seborrhoeic*: greasy debris around the lashes causing them to adhere to one another (Fig. 2)
- *Posterior*: frothy tear film (Fig. 3) and plugging of the meibomian gland orifices (Fig. 4)

All types usually manifest hyperaemia of the lid margins (Fig. 5) and conjunctiva, and tear film instability.

Complications

Corneal epitheliopathy, scarring, and marginal keratitis (see Fig. 102); recurrent bacterial conjunctivitis, chalazia (see Fig. 7) and styes (see Fig.10). Loss of lashes (madarosis) and misdirection (trichiasis; Fig. 6).

Management

- Lid margin hygiene using a weak solution of baby shampoo
- Tear substitutes (e.g. hypromellose, carbomers)
- Antibiotic ointment (e.g. fusidic acid, chloramphenicol) rubbed into the lid margins
- Systemic tetracycline.

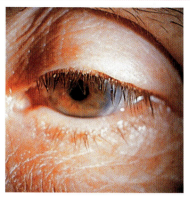

Fig. 1 Scales around eyelash bases in staphylococcal anterior blepharitis.

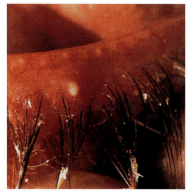

Fig. 2 Greasy adherent lashes, in seborrhoeic posterior blepharitis.

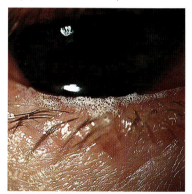

Fig. 3 Foam in the tear film.

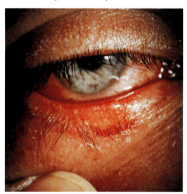

Fig. 4 Blocked meibomian gland orifices in posterior blepharitis.

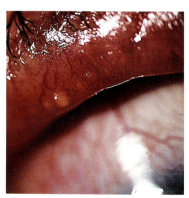

Fig. 5 Hyperaemia of lid margin.

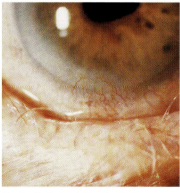

Fig. 6 Eyelash misdirection in long-standing anterior blepharitis.

2 Non-neoplastic eyelid nodules

Meibomian cyst (chalazion)

Definition
A lesion consisting of lipogranulomatous inflammation centred on a dysfunctional meibomian gland.

Clinical features
Extremely common, particularly in patients with posterior blepharitis. A chronic, usually solitary, painless, firm swelling in the tarsal plate (Fig. 7); can follow an acute meibomian gland infection (see below). May be associated with a secondary conjunctival granuloma (Fig. 8).

Management
Spontaneous resolution may occur, although usually only if the lesion is small. Surgical incision and curettage is often required.

Internal hordeolum (acute chalazion)

Definition
An acute bacterial meibomian gland infection.

Clinical features
An inflamed swelling within the tarsal plate which may be associated with preseptal cellulitis (Fig. 9).

Management
Topical antibiotic ointment and systemic antibiotics (e.g. flucloxacillin) for preseptal cellulitis. Hot bathing may promote discharge. Incision and curettage may be required for a large abscess, or for a secondary chronic lesion.

External hordeolum (stye)

Definition
A small abscess of an eyelash follicle.

Clinical features
An acute, painful inflamed swelling on the anterior lid margin, usually pointing through the skin (Fig. 10).

Management
Removal of the associated lash, and hot bathing. Topical antibiotic ointment. Large lesions may require incision.

Cysts of Zeis and Moll

Clinical features
A cyst of Zeis is a small, whitish, chronic, painless, opaque nodule on the lid margin (Fig. 11). A cyst of Moll is similar but translucent.

Management
Simple excision.

Molluscum contagiosum

Clinical features
Single or multiple, small, pale, waxy umbilicated nodules (Fig. 12), which may cause a secondary chronic ipsilateral follicular conjunctivitis (see Fig. 55). These virally transmitted lesions are common and more severe in AIDS patients.

Management
Expression or cautery.

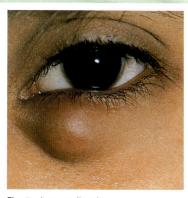

Fig. 7 Large meibomian cyst.

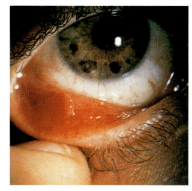

Fig. 8 Conjunctival granuloma secondary to meibomian cyst.

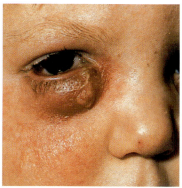

Fig. 9 Internal hordeolum with preseptal cellulitis.

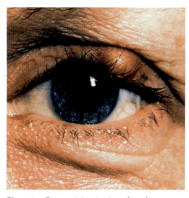

Fig. 10 External hordeolum (stye).

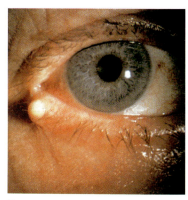

Fig. 11 Cyst of Zeis.

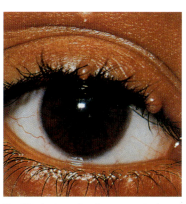

Fig. 12 Lesions of molluscum contagiosum.

3 Benign tumours of the eyelids

Squamous cell papilloma (viral wart)

Clinical features

The most common benign tumour of the eyelid which may be broad-based (sessile) or pedunculated (Fig. 13).

Management

Simple excision, cautery or laser ablation.

Basal cell papilloma (seborrhoeic keratosis)

Clinical features

This common tumour, usually found in the elderly, is a slowly-enlarging brownish papillary lesion with a greasy, friable surface (Fig. 14).

Management

Simple excision or curettage.

Keratoacanthoma

Clinical features

An uncommon, fast-growing, firm, pinkish nodule that develops a keratin-filled crater (Fig. 15) and may be mistaken for a malignancy. Remains static for several months before undergoing spontaneous involution.

Melanocytic naevus

Intradermal naevus An elevated lesion with variable pigmentation. When located on the lid margin may be associated with protruding lashes (Fig. 16). No malignant potential.

Junctional naevus A flat, well circumscribed lesion with a uniform brown colour, so-called because the naevus cells are located at the junction of the dermis and epidermis. Low malignant potential.

Compound naevus Usually elevated, with a homogeneous tan to brown colour. Consists of both intradermal and junctional components, the latter conferring a low malignant potential.

Capillary haemangioma (strawberry naevus)

Clinical features

An irregular red lesion in an infant which may cause a mechanical ptosis and amblyopia (Fig. 17).

Management

Local steroids if necessary, but frequently undergoes gradual spontaneous involution.

Plexiform neurofibroma

Typically occurs in neurofibromatosis-1, characteristically giving rise to an S-shaped lid margin and ptosis (Fig. 18).

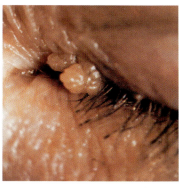

Fig. 13 Squamous cell papilloma (viral wart).

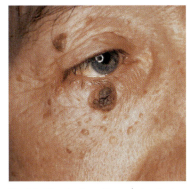

Fig. 14 Basal cell papilloma (seborrhoeic keratosis).

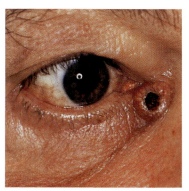

Fig. 15 Keratoacanthoma.

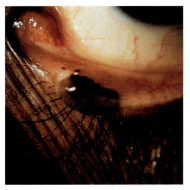

Fig. 16 Intradermal naevus.

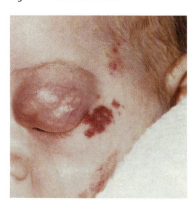

Fig. 17 Capillary haemangioma (strawberry naevus).

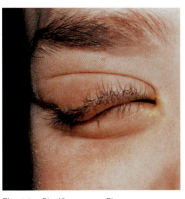

Fig. 18 Plexiform neurofibroma.

4 Premalignant and malignant tumours of the eyelids

Actinic (solar) keratosis

Clinical features

Although rare, this is the most common premalignant lid condition and is strongly associated with excessive sun exposure in light-skinned individuals. It usually presents as a persistent scaly plaque (Fig. 19), which must be biopsied.

Basal cell carcinoma

Basal cell carcinoma (BCC), the most common eyelid malignancy, is locally invasive but does not metastasize. About 50% involve the lower lid, 30% the medial canthal area.

Clinical features

Nodulo-ulcerative A 'rodent ulcer', with rolled hyperkeratotic edges and central granulation (Fig. 20), gradually enlarging over 1–2 years. A purely nodular appearance is common (Fig. 21).

Sclerosing A flat indurated plaque with poorly demarcated margins, often with loss of overlying lashes (Fig. 22).

Squamous cell carcinoma

Clinical features

Squamous cell carcinoma (SCC) is much less common than BCC. It grows more quickly and may metastasize. It may arise de novo or from a premalignant condition such as actinic keratosis (see above).

Nodular SCC Starts as a hyperkeratotic nodule or plaque which later develops crusting fissures.

Ulcerative SCC Resembles a rodent ulcer (Fig. 23).

Sebaceous gland carcinoma

Clinical features

This is a rare but very aggressive tumour, which may originate in a meibomian or Zeis gland as a firm nodule either on the lid margin or within the tarsal plate (Fig. 24), when it may be mistaken for a chalazion (see Fig. 7).

Management

- Surgical excision with a wide clearance margin is the treatment of choice for most lid malignancies
- Radiotherapy in selected cases.

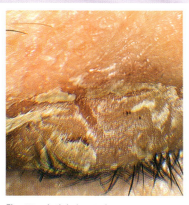

Fig. 19 Actinic keratosis.

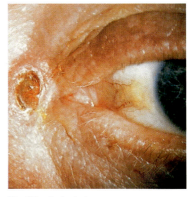

Fig. 20 Rodent ulcer.

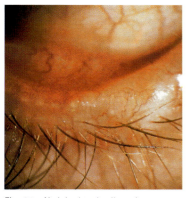

Fig. 21 Nodular basal cell carcinoma.

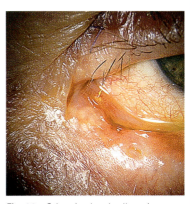

Fig. 22 Sclerosing basal cell carcinoma.

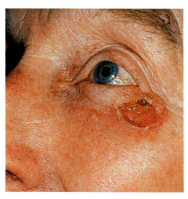

Fig. 23 Ulcerative squamous cell carcinoma.

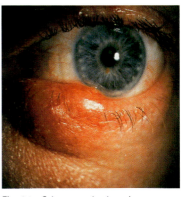

Fig. 24 Sebaceous gland carcinoma.

5 Ptosis

Definition	The upper eyelid rests at a lower position than normal.

Classification

Neurogenic
- *Third (oculomotor) nerve palsy* (Fig. 25): must exclude 'surgical' cause (e.g. aneurysm, tumour) compressing nerve
- *Horner's syndrome* (Fig. 26): congenital or acquired dysfunction of the sympathetic autonomic pathway
- *Marcus Gunn ('jaw-winking') syndrome*: congenital, uncommon.

Aponeurotic
- *Involutional*: age-related laxity of the levator aponeurosis (Fig. 27)
- *Postoperative*: stretching of the aponeurosis during surgery.

Mechanical
- *Excessive lid weight*: oedema, tumours (see Figs 17, 18), redundant skin
- *Cicatricial*: reduced mobility from scarring of the upper lid skin or conjunctiva.

Myogenic
- *Simple congenital*: unilateral or bilateral (Fig. 28)
- *Blepharophimosis syndrome*: rare, congenital bilateral ptosis, associated with other eyelid and facial abnormalities (Fig. 29)
- *Acquired*: myasthenia gravis, ocular myopathy, myotonic dystrophy (Fig. 30).

Salient points

- *Third nerve palsy*: pupillary involvement carries high index of suspicion for 'surgical' aetiology. Misdirection of regenerating nerve fibres may occur, resulting in ptosis or lid retraction on eye movement
- *Horner's syndrome*: ipsilateral miosis, heterochromia if congenital, sweating decreased on affected side dependent on location of lesion.

Management

- Address any treatable cause (e.g. myasthenia gravis)
- Surgical options include levator or aponeurosis strengthening and frontalis (brow) suspension.

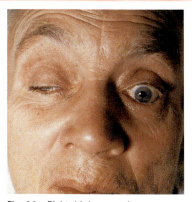

Fig. 26   Right third nerve palsy.

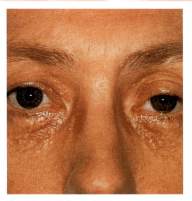

Fig. 26   Left Horner's syndrome.

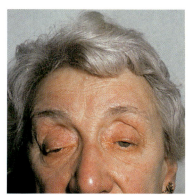

Fig. 27   Severe bilateral involutional ptosis.

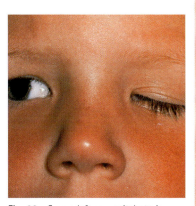

Fig. 28   Severe left congenital ptosis.

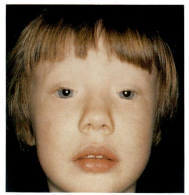

Fig. 29   Blepharophimosis syndrome.

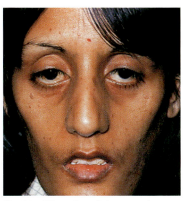

Fig. 30   Bilateral ptosis in myotonic dystrophy.

6 Entropion, ectropion and trichiasis

Entropion

Definition
An inward-turning of the eyelid. If severe or prolonged may cause corneal scarring (Fig. 31).

Classification
- *Involutional*: most common form; results from age-related changes in the lower lid
- *Cicatricial*: most frequently secondary to scarring of the upper palpebral conjunctiva, as in chronic trachoma (Fig. 32)
- *Spastic*: lower lid; caused by spasm of the orbicularis muscle due to ocular irritation or essential blepharospasm. Frequently temporary
- *Congenital*: very rare; only involves the lower lid. Caused by hypertrophy of skin and orbicularis.

Management
Surgical correction.

Ectropion

Definition
An outward-turning eyelid, virtually exclusively involving the lower lid. If severe and prolonged may cause conjunctival keratinization (Fig. 33).

Classification
- *Involutional*: the most common form; age-related tissue laxity
- *Cicatricial*: scarring resulting from burns or surgery (e.g. tumour resection; Fig. 34)
- *Mechanical*: excess lid weight (e.g. large tumour)
- *Paralytic*: facial nerve palsy; associated with incomplete blinking and lid closure (Fig. 35)
- *Congenital*: may be part of the blepharophimosis syndrome (see Fig. 29).

Management
Surgical correction.

Trichiasis

Definition
Inward misdirection of lashes, often secondary to acute or chronic lid inflammation (e.g. blepharitis, trachoma). Typically causes corneal irritation and sometimes scarring (Fig. 36). Should be differentiated from distichiasis, in which extra lashes (usually congenital) arise from meibomian gland orifices.

Management
Options include simple epilation, electrolysis, cryotherapy and laser ablation.

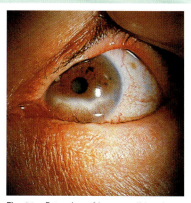

Fig. 31 Entropion of lower eyelid and corneal scarring.

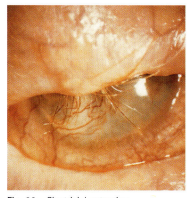

Fig. 32 Cicatricial entropion.

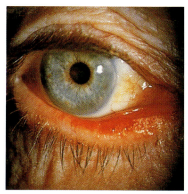

Fig. 33 Ectropion and conjunctival keratinization.

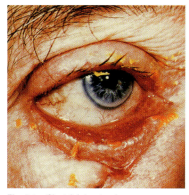

Fig. 34 Cicatricial ectropion.

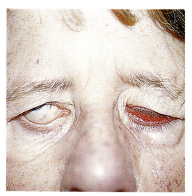

Fig. 35 Paralytic ectropian with poor lid closure.

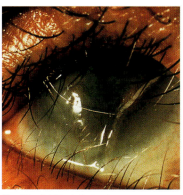

Fig. 36 Trichiasis in trachoma.

Aetiology

Autoantibodies to both thyroid and orbital tissue cause inflammation; the extraocular muscles are particularly affected.

Clinical features

The clinical course involves an 'active' congestive stage, usually lasting 2–3 years, followed by a 'quiescent' stage in which residual restriction of ocular movements may be the chief feature.

Symptoms
- Redness
- Irritation
- Aching
- Wide-eyed 'staring' appearance
- Double vision
- Decreased vision in severe cases.

Signs
- Fullness of the eyelids
- Conjunctival hyperaemia and chemosis (Fig. 37)
- Proptosis (exophthalmos): may be unilateral or bilateral (Fig. 38). If severe, may prevent adequate lid closure with resultant exposure keratopathy
- Lid retraction in primary position (Fig. 39), which compounds the cosmetic effect of proptosis
- Lid lag in downgaze (von Graefe's sign)
- Ophthalmoplegia due to inflammation early in the disease and subsequently to fibrosis. The inferior and medial recti are most frequently affected
- Choroidal folds (Fig. 40)
- Optic neuropathy is a sight-threatening complication caused by compression of the optic nerve or its blood supply by swollen orbital tissue, particularly extraocular muscles. Useful tests include colour vision, visual acuity and visual fields. There may be a relative afferent pupillary defect and optic disc oedema.

Management
- Tear substitutes and topical steroids for conjunctival and corneal involvement
- Systemic steroids are usually reserved for optic neuropathy
- Surgery for proptosis (orbital decompression), diplopia (muscle surgery) and eyelid retraction
- Radiotherapy may be appropriate for the congestive phase, if severe.

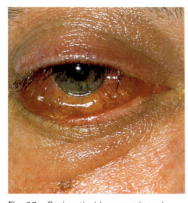

Fig. 37 Conjunctival hyperaemia and chemosis.

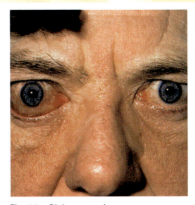

Fig. 38 Right proptosis.

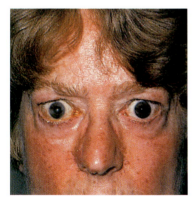

Fig. 39 Bilateral lid retraction.

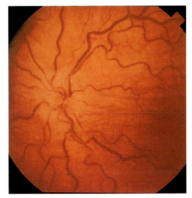

Fig. 40 Choroidal folds.

Capillary haemangioma

Clinical features

Presents in infancy with an anterior orbital swelling (Fig. 41), which may increase in size when crying. A similar eyelid skin lesion, a 'strawberry naevus' (see Fig. 17), may also be present.

Management

Steroids injected into the lesion or given systemically are effective but the tumour often involutes spontaneously.

Cavernous haemangioma

Clinical features

The most common benign orbital tumour in adults. Presents in young adults with painless axial proptosis of gradual onset.

Management

Surgical excision.

Orbital varices

Clinical features

Dilated orbital veins. Presentation is at any age with:
- Intermittent unilateral non-pulsatile proptosis
- Visible lesions in the eyelids or conjunctiva (Fig. 42)
- Acute orbital haemorrhage or thrombosis (less common).

Management

Surgical excision may be required.

Rhabdomyosarcoma

Clinical features

This very rare but aggressive tumour typically presents at about the age of 7 years with progressive proptosis and a palpable mass may be present (Fig. 43).

Management

Incisional biopsy followed by radiotherapy and chemotherapy.

Neural tumours

Optic nerve glioma   Presents in childhood with slowly progressive proptosis and visual loss. The optic disc may be swollen or pale (see Fig. 238). 25–50% of patients have neurofibromatosis-1.

Optic nerve sheath meningioma   Typically affects middle-aged females and causes slowly progressive visual loss followed later by proptosis (Fig. 44). The optic disc frequently shows opticociliary shunt vessels (Fig. 45).

Management

Options include observation, surgery and radiotherapy.

Dermoid cyst

Clinical features

Variable age at presentation, with proptosis and/or a palpable mass (Fig. 46) depending on site and size.

Management

Excision, which must be complete.

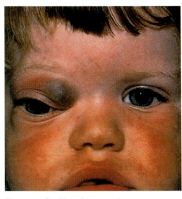

Fig. 41 Capillary haemangioma.

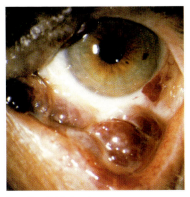

Fig. 42 Orbital varices.

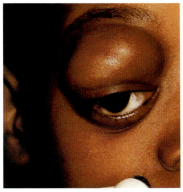

Fig. 43 Rhabdomyosarcoma.

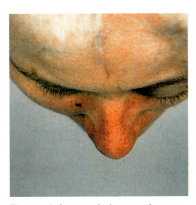

Fig. 44 Left proptosis due to optic nerve sheath meningioma.

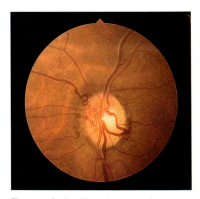

Fig. 45 Opticociliary shunt vessels.

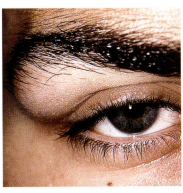

Fig. 46 Dermoid cyst.

9 Miscellaneous orbital disease

Orbital cellulitis

Definition A potentially life-threatening acute bacterial infection of the soft tissues of the orbit.

Aetiology
- Secondary to sinusitis (usually in children)
- Spread from infected adjacent structures (e.g. dacryocystitis)
- Following trauma and surgery.

Clinical features

Symptoms Acute lid swelling and redness, pain and malaise.

Signs Reduced visual acuity, lid oedema and erythema (Fig. 47), chemosis, proptosis, painful ophthalmoplegia and optic disc swelling.

Complications Intracranial infection, cavernous sinus thrombosis, subperiosteal abscess, and blindness.

Management
- Intravenous antibiotics
- Orbital CT, principally to rule out an abscess
- Surgery for abscess drainage or sinus washout.

Idiopathic orbital inflammation (pseudotumour)

Definition Idiopathic inflammation of the soft tissues of the orbit.

Clinical features Subacute onset of unilateral pain, lid oedema, chemosis, proptosis (Fig. 48), decreased vision and ophthalmoplegia.

Management Systemic steroids, radiotherapy or cytotoxic agents.

Carotid–cavernous fistula

Definition Indirect or direct arterial communication with the cavernous sinus. Usually due to trauma or spontaneous arterial rupture.

Clinical features Headache, chemosis (Fig. 49), dilated episcleral vessels (Fig. 50), pulsatile proptosis with associated thrill and bruit, ophthalmoplegia, raised intraocular pressure and retinal vascular congestion and haemorrhages (Fig. 51).

Management Radiological intervention if appropriate.

Blow-out fracture of orbital floor

Clinical features Periorbital oedema and ecchymosis, enophthalmos (Fig. 52), vertical diplopia, infraorbital nerve anaesthesia and subcutaneous emphysema.

Management Surgery may be necessary in severe cases.

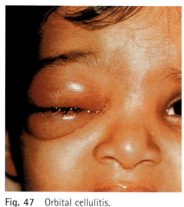

Fig. 47 Orbital cellulitis.

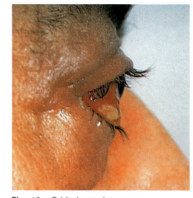

Fig. 48 Orbital pseudotumour.

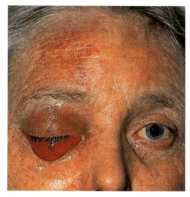

Fig. 49 Severe chemosis due to direct carotid–cavernous fistula.

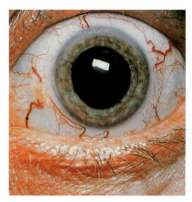

Fig. 50 Dilated episcleral vessels due to indirect carotid–cavernous fistula.

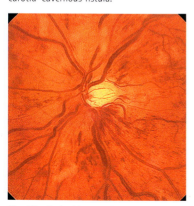

Fig. 51 Retinal haemorrhages and dilated veins in carotid–cavernous fistula.

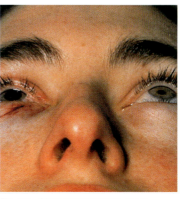

Fig. 52 Right enophthalmos due to orbital floor blow-out fracture.

Acute allergic conjunctivitis

Acute onset of bilateral itching, lid oedema and chemosis (Fig. 53), often in children after playing on grass in spring or summer. Settles spontaneously within a few hours.

Seasonal allergic (hay fever) conjunctivitis

Clinical features
Persistent itching, conjunctival hyperaemia and excess mucus production during the hay fever season.

Management
Topical mast cell stabilizers and antihistamines usually provide adequate symptomatic relief.

Bacterial conjunctivitis

Clinical features
Subacute onset of bilateral, but frequently asymmetrical, redness, grittiness and a sticky discharge. Examination shows conjunctival hyperaemia (Fig. 54) and mild papillary changes. Visual acuity, corneas and pupils are normal.

Management
Topical antibiotics (e.g. chloramphenicol, fusidic acid, gentamicin) for about a week.

Adenoviral conjunctivitis

Clinical features
Acute onset of frequently bilateral grittiness and redness and a watery discharge. Examination shows a follicular conjunctival reaction (Fig. 55), preauricular lymphadenopathy, lid oedema, chemosis and subconjunctival haemorrhages (Fig. 56). A punctate epithelial keratitis may progress to persistent deeper infiltrates (Fig. 57). The condition is highly contagious.

Management
Topical lubricants; steroids may be considered for severe keratitis.

Neonatal conjunctivitis

Definition
A conjunctival inflammation occurring within the first month of life.

Aetiology
The timing of presentation may aid diagnosis.
- *Chlamydia*: the most common (Fig. 58); presents at 1–3 weeks
- *Gonococcus*: during first week
- *Herpes simplex*: 1–2 weeks
- *Simple bacterial conjunctivitis*: end of first week onwards.

Management
- Ensure cornea is uninvolved
- Investigate and treat individual conditions as appropriate (including maternal infection).

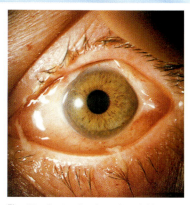

Fig. 53 Acute allergic conjunctivitis.

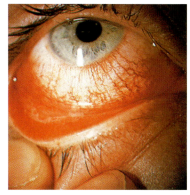

Fig. 54 Bacterial conjunctivitis.

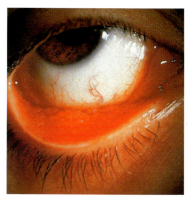

Fig. 55 Follicular conjunctivitis in adenoviral infection.

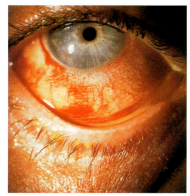

Fig. 56 Subconjunctival haemorrhages in severe adenoviral conjunctivitis.

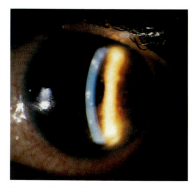

Fig. 57 Corneal infiltrates following adenoviral conjunctivitis.

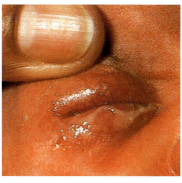

Fig. 58 Mucopurulent discharge in neonatal chlamydial infection.

11 Chronic conjunctivitis

Adult chlamydial conjunctivitis

Clinical features

Sexually transmitted infection presenting with subacute onset of typically unilateral mucopurulent discharge associated with large conjunctival follicles (Fig. 59) and preauricular lymphadenopathy.

Management

- Laboratory testing to confirm diagnosis
- Referral for assessment by a genitourinary specialist
- Treat with antibiotics (e.g. azithromycin).

Vernal keratoconjunctivitis (VKC)

Clinical features

A bilateral chronic or recurrent allergic condition that starts in childhood, usually in patients with atopy (e.g. asthma, eczema and hay fever).

Symptoms include itching, watering, photophobia and a stringy discharge. Papillary conjunctivitis particularly involves the superior tarsus (Fig. 60) and sometimes the limbus (Fig. 61). Corneal signs include punctate epitheliopathy, ulceration, plaque formation (Fig. 62) and scarring, occasionally in the form of a limbal 'Cupid's bow' ('pseudogerontoxon' – Fig. 63).

Management

Topical mast cell stabilizers, antihistamines and topical steroids.

Atopic keratoconjunctivitis

Clinical features

A rare condition typically affecting young men with atopic dermatitis (eczema). Similar to VKC but carries a worse prognosis. The eyelids are thickened and crusted, and associated staphylococcal blepharitis (see Fig. 1) is common. Intense papillary conjunctivitis may lead to symblepharon (see Fig. 75), and corneal complications can be severe. Aggressive herpes simplex keratitis (see Fig. 86) and microbial keratitis (see Figs 77–80) may occur.

Management

Similar to VKC but frequently more resistant.

Giant papillary conjunctivitis

A foreign-body-associated conjunctivitis characterized by giant papillae on the superior tarsus (Fig. 64). Causes include contact lens wear, artificial eyes and protruding sutures.

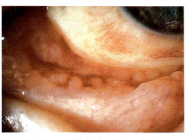

Fig. 59   Large follicles in chlamydial conjunctivitis.

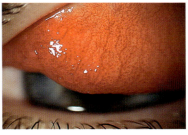

Fig. 60   Papillary conjunctivitis.

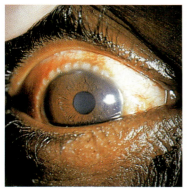

Fig. 61   Vernal limbitis.

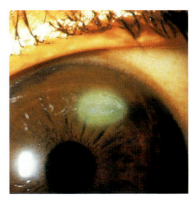

Fig. 62   Corneal plaque.

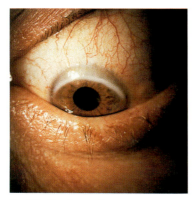

Fig. 63   Pseudogerontoxon.

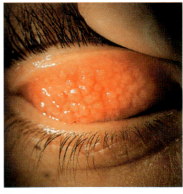

Fig. 64   Giant papillae.

12 Conjunctival tumours

Papilloma

Pedunculated papilloma Caused by a papillomavirus. Typically affects children and young adults and may be multiple. Usually located on the palpebral conjunctiva, fornix or caruncle.

Sessile papilloma Affects older patients. Invariably single and unilateral (Fig. 65), located on the bulbar conjunctiva or at the limbus.

Carcinoma

Conjunctival and corneal intra-epithelial neoplasia (CCIN) A slightly elevated, fleshy vascular or gelatinous mobile mass, most frequently juxtalimbal (Fig. 66), sometimes with corneal extension. Low malignant potential.

Invasive carcinoma Similar in appearance but fixed to underlying tissues.

Choristoma

Dermoid A rounded, white nodule typically located at the limbus (Fig. 67).

Lipodermoid A soft yellow-white subconjunctival mass usually found at the outer canthus.

Pigmented lesions

Conjunctival (racial) epithelial melanosis A very common physiological pigmentation in dark-skinned individuals.

Conjunctival naevus An uncommon lesion presenting during childhood or early adult life. Single, well-demarcated, flat or slightly elevated, variably pigmented lesion, most commonly at the limbus (Fig. 68); size/pigmentation may increase at puberty.

Primary acquired melanosis (PAM) A rare condition presenting in old age with uni- or multifocal slowly growing patches of intraepithelial pigmentation. Some malignant potential.

Melanoma A rare tumour accounting for 2% of all ocular malignancies. Most frequently arises within PAM, as a nodular lesion (Fig. 69). May arise from a pre-existing naevus or, rarely, de novo, usually at the limbus (Fig. 70).

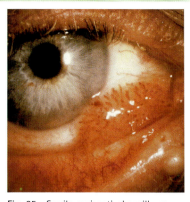

Fig. 65   Sessile conjunctival papilloma.

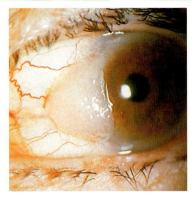

Fig. 66   Conjunctival and corneal intraepithelial neoplasia.

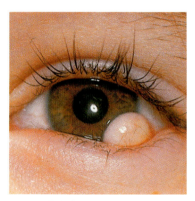

Fig. 67   Limbal dermoid.

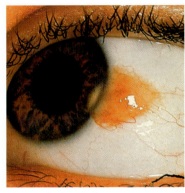

Fig. 68   Conjunctival naevus.

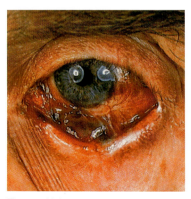

Fig. 69   Melanoma arising within an area of primary acquired melanosis.

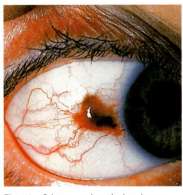

Fig. 70   Primary conjunctival melanoma.

Keratoconjunctivitis sicca

Aetiology

Keratoconjunctivitis sicca (KCS), or 'dry eye', is a very common condition resulting from any process that affects the production or evaporation of the tears. Age-related lacrimal gland atrophy and autoimmune damage (Sjögren's syndrome) are common causes; secondary Sjögren's syndrome is the association of KCS with a connective tissue disorder (e.g. rheumatoid arthritis).

Clinical features

Symptoms Include grittiness and redness, often worse in the evening.

Signs
- Irregular patchy tear film with rapid break-up after blinking
- Thin marginal tear strip with mucous debris
- Dry conjunctiva and cornea stains with Rose Bengal (Fig. 71)
- Corneal filaments (Fig. 72)
- Schirmer's test measures the wetting of a strip of filter paper: typically reduced.

Management
- Tear substitutes usually suffice if used regularly
- Punctal occlusion in severe cases.

Cicatrizing conjunctivitis

Aetiology

Bilateral conjunctival manifestation of immune-mediated blistering mucocutaneous diseases; serious but rare.

Cicatricial pemphigoid A chronic disease characterized by skin and mucous membrane blister formation.

Stevens–Johnson syndrome An acute, severe but generally self-limiting vasculitis most commonly caused by hypersensitivity to certain drugs and infections. Characteristic 'target' skin lesions and oral mucosal lesions (Fig. 73) are seen.

Complications
- Conjunctival scarring (Fig. 74) and shrinkage
- Adhesions between the bulbar and palpebral conjunctiva (symblepharon, Fig. 75), and of the outer canthi (ankyloblepharon)
- Dry eye
- Aberrant eyelash growth
- Cicatricial entropion
- Corneal keratinization (Fig. 76).

Management
- Topical and systemic steroids
- Tear substitutes
- Surgery (mainly for lid deformity).

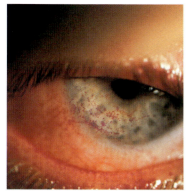

Fig. 71 Dry conjunctiva and cornea stained with Rose Bengal.

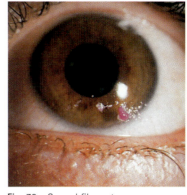

Fig. 72 Corneal filaments.

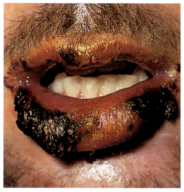

Fig. 73 Haemorrhagic crusting of lips in Stevens–Johnson syndrome.

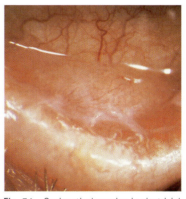

Fig. 74 Conjunctival scarring in cicatricial pemphigoid.

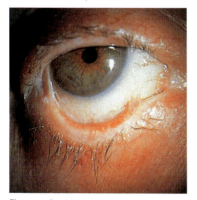

Fig. 75 Symblepharon.

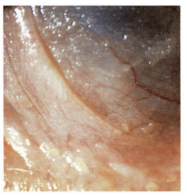

Fig. 76 Corneal keratinization in cicatricial pemphigoid.

Bacterial keratitis

Clinical features

This serious condition is usually associated with pre-existing corneal surface disease or contact lens wear.

Symptoms Subacute onset of unilateral pain, redness, photophobia and blurred vision

Signs Circumcorneal injection, stromal infiltrate and an overlying epithelial defect. A hypopyon may be present if severe.

Aetiology

Staphylococcal and pneumococcal typically causes yellow-white, oval suppuration surrounded by relatively clear cornea (Figs 77, 78).

Pseudomonas causes irregular suppuration associated with a mucopurulent discharge (Figs 79, 80). Very severe infections may extend into the sclera.

Management

Specimens for culture (corneal scrape, conjunctival swab, contact lenses/case if available) followed by intensive topical antibiotics (e.g. ofloxacin, fortified cefuroxime/gentamicin combination).

Fungal keratitis

Clinical features

Filamentous Frequently preceded by ocular trauma involving vegetable matter. Characterized by greyish-white ulceration with indistinct feathery margins and satellite lesions (Fig. 81).

Candida Typically occurs in debilitated patients or those with pre-existing surface disease; similar appearance to bacterial keratitis.

Management Topical antifungal agents.

Acanthamoeba keratitis

Clinical features

Patients, usually contact lens wearers, typically experience pain disproportionate to the clinical signs. Early cases are characterized by dendritiform epithelial lesions, radial keratoneuritis and stromal keratitis followed by a central ring abscess associated with variable epithelial breakdown (Fig. 82).

Management Topical amoebicidal agents.

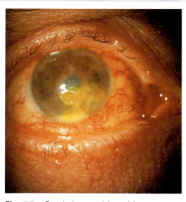

Fig. 77 Staphylococcal keratitis.

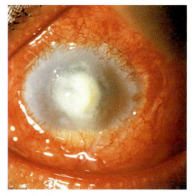

Fig. 78 Pneumococcal keratitis.

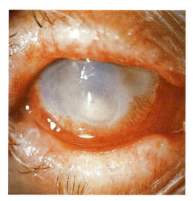

Fig. 79 Pseudomonas keratitis.

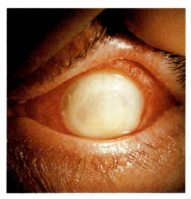

Fig. 80 Advanced pseudomonas keratitis.

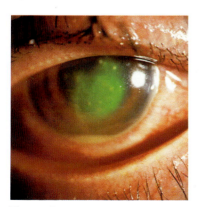

Fig. 81 Fungal keratitis.

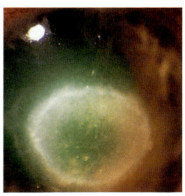

Fig. 82 Acanthamoeba keratitis.

Primary infection

This is caused by direct transmission of virus through infected secretions to a non-immune subject, usually a child. It may cause follicular conjunctivitis (see Fig. 55), blepharitis (Fig. 83) and epithelial keratitis.

Recurrent epithelial keratitis

Aetiology

Invasion of the corneal epithelium by reactivated latent virus; common.

Clinical features

Corneal sensation is diminished. A branching 'dendritic' ulcer is characteristic, demonstrated well with fluorescein staining (Fig. 84). A geographical (amoeboid) ulcer (Fig. 85) develops from an enlarging dendritic lesion particularly when the latter has inadvertently been treated with topical steroids.

Management

Topical antiviral agents (e.g. aciclovir, ganciclovir).

Stromal necrotic keratitis

Aetiology

This uncommon condition is caused by direct viral invasion and destruction of the corneal stroma.

Clinical features

Cheesy, necrotic stroma appearing similar to bacterial or fungal infection (Fig. 86), with associated anterior uveitis. Complications include scarring (Fig. 87) and perforation.

Management

- Treatment of any associated epithelial defect
- Topical steroids, to reduce stromal inflammation, with antiviral and antibiotic cover.

Disciform keratitis

Aetiology

Possibly a hypersensitivity reaction to herpes virus.

Clinical features

Subacute, usually painless blurring of vision which may be associated with haloes around lights. Examination shows an area of epithelial and stromal oedema with associated keratic precipitates (Fig. 88). Other findings include mild iritis and a ring of infiltrates surrounding the lesion (Wessely ring).

Management

Topical steroids combined with antiviral cover. In some cases, oral aciclovir may be considered to reduce recurrence.

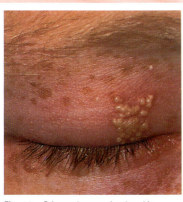

Fig. 83 Primary herpes simplex skin lesions.

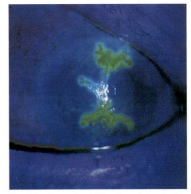

Fig. 84 Large dendritic ulcer stained with fluorescein.

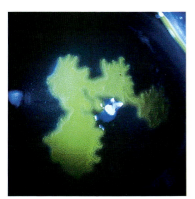

Fig. 85 Geographical herpetic ulcer stained with fluorescein.

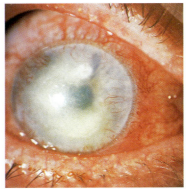

Fig. 86 Stromal necrotic keratitis.

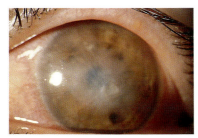

Fig. 87 Scarring complicating stromal keratitis.

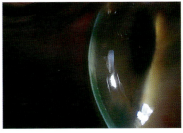

Fig. 88 Disciform keratitis.

Aetiology	Herpes zoster (shingles) is caused by the varicella zoster virus.
Definition	Approximately 15% of all cases of herpes zoster affect the ophthalmic division of the trigeminal nerve (herpes zoster ophthalmicus).
Clinical features	**Skin lesions** An initial maculopapular rash evolves to form vesicles (small blisters), which subsequently burst to form crusting ulcers. Periorbital oedema is common (Fig. 89). Postherpetic neuralgia can be severe, chronic and very distressing.

Ocular complications
Ocular involvement is common when the rash involves the side of the nose (Hutchinson's sign).

- *Conjunctivitis and episcleritis*: very common and usually transient
- *Acute iritis*: common and may give rise to elevation of intraocular pressure and segmental iris atrophy (Fig. 90)
- *Acute keratitis*: punctate epithelial, filamentary (see Fig. 72), microdendritic, nummular (Fig. 91) and disciform (see Fig. 88)
- *Chronic corneal lesions*: mucus plaque keratitis, secondary lipid keratopathy (Fig. 92) and neurotrophic keratitis, which may lead to extreme thinning (Fig. 93) and perforation
- *Scleritis* (Fig. 94): uncommon and frequently involves the cornea (sclerokeratitis)
- *Neuro-ophthalmological*: optic neuritis and extraocular muscle palsies.

Management	

- If administered early, systemic antiviral agents (e.g. aciclovir, valaciclovir, famciclovir) curtail the rash and reduce ocular complications and neuralgia
- Steroid–antibiotic preparations (e.g. hydrocortisone–fusidic acid) applied to the skin may be beneficial prior to crust separation
- Treatment of iritis and most acute corneal lesions is with topical steroids.

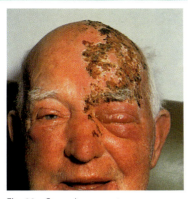

Fig. 89 Severe herpes zoster ophthalmicus.

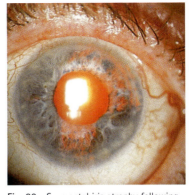

Fig. 90 Segmental iris atrophy following herpes zoster iritis.

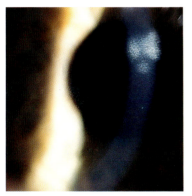

Fig. 91 Nummular keratitis.

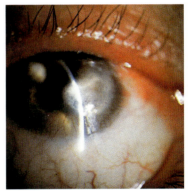

Fig. 92 Lipid keratopathy.

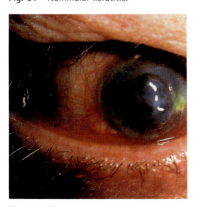

Fig. 93 Severe corneal thinning.

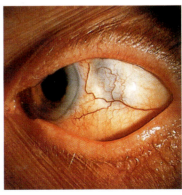

Fig. 94 Scleral thinning due to previous scleritis.

17 Corneal dystrophies

Clinical features

Epithelial basement membrane (Cogan microcystic or map–dot–fingerprint) dystrophy

Common, sporadic and non-progressive. Presents in second or third decade with recurrent corneal erosions characterized by grittiness, lacrimation and photophobia on waking. Examination shows subtle bilateral dot-like, cystic (Fig. 95) or linear epithelial lesions.

Reis–Bücklers and Thiel-Behnke dystrophies

Presentation of these dominantly inherited dystrophies of the Bowman layer, which underlies the corneal epithelium, is during the first decade of life with recurrent corneal erosions, followed later by variable blurring of vision. Bilateral superficial reticular or honeycomb-pattern opacities are seen (Fig. 96).

Lattice dystrophies

This group (types 1–3) of rare, dominantly inherited dystrophies presents at varying ages with recurrent corneal erosions. On examination a network of spidery lines involves the anterior and mid stroma (Fig. 97), the precise morphology being dependent on type.

Granular dystrophy

Rare, dominantly inherited, presenting during the first decade with recurrent erosions. Discrete, crumb-like granules are seen within the anterior stroma (Fig. 98).

Fuchs' endothelial dystrophy

Presentation of this, usually sporadic condition, is in later life with initially unilateral visual impairment. Examination shows corneal oedema – 'bullous keratopathy' if severe (Fig. 99). The fellow eye invariably shows characteristic endothelial changes (cornea guttata).

Management

- Varies according to type and severity of dystrophy
- Lubricants alone in mild cases
- Bandage contact lenses for severe erosions and painful bullous keratopathy
- Corneal grafting (Fig. 100) for advanced disease.

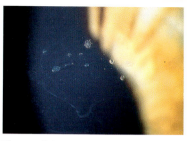

Fig. 95 Epithelial basement membrane dystrophy.

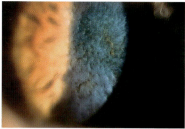

Fig. 96 Honeycomb opacities in Thiel–Behnke dystrophy.

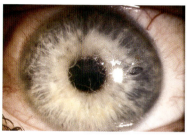

Fig. 97 Lattice dystrophy.

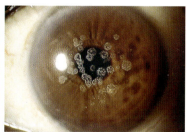

Fig. 98 Granular dystrophy.

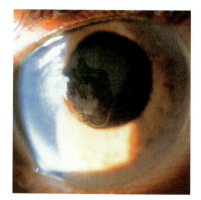

Fig. 99 Bullous keratopathy.

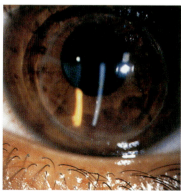

Fig. 100 Corneal graft (penetrating keratoplasty).

Dellen

Clinical features

An area of thinning secondary to local stromal dehydration, most frequently associated with an elevated limbal lesion (Fig. 101).

Management

Eliminate the cause and promote rehydration by patching and lubricants.

Marginal keratitis

Aetiology

Hypersensitivity to staphylococcal exotoxins. Very common and frequently associated with chronic anterior blepharitis (see Fig. 1).

Clinical features

Subepithelial infiltrate, separated from the limbus by clear cornea (Fig. 102), often with an overlying smaller area of epithelial breakdown.

Management

Short course of topical steroids (e.g. fluorometholone, prednisolone 0.5%).

Rosacea keratitis

Clinical features

Occurs in about 5% of patients with acne rosacea. Inferior punctate epitheliopathy that may progress to subepithelial infiltration and peripheral vascularization (Fig. 103). Occasionally severe peripheral thinning and perforation may occur.

Management

- Topical steroids
- Systemic tetracycline or doxycycline.

Ulceration associated with rheumatoid arthritis

Clinical features

May be chronic, without inflammation (Fig. 104) or acute and associated with severe inflammation at the limbus (Fig. 105).

Management

- Lubricants
- Topical and systemic steroids
- Other systemic immunosuppressants.

Mooren's ulcer

Clinical features

Very rare but serious, painful condition that may be unilateral or bilateral and may spread circumferentially or centrally (Fig. 106).

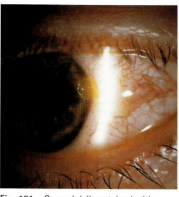

Fig. 101 Corneal dellen stained with fluorescein.

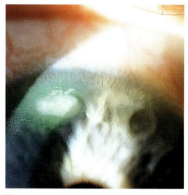

Fig. 102 Marginal keratitis.

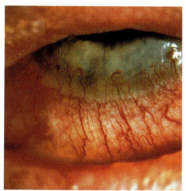

Fig. 103 Rosacea keratitis.

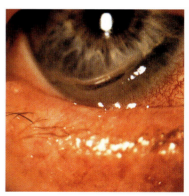

Fig. 104 Corneal melting in rheumatoid arthritis.

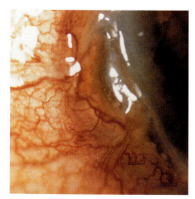

Fig. 105 Acute corneal ulceration in rheumatoid arthritis.

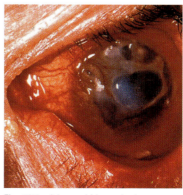

Fig. 106 Advanced Mooren's ulcer.

19 Disorders of corneal size and shape

Keratoconus

Clinical features

Fairly common cone-like bulging of the central cornea (Fig. 107), presenting during the second or third decades of life with slowly progressive blurring of vision from irregular astigmatism. Both eyes are affected in almost all cases, though often asymmetrically.

Early signs   Include abnormal ophthalmoscopy reflex, irregular 'scissors' retinoscopy reflex and fine vertical lines in the deep stroma (Vogt striae – Fig. 108).

Late signs   Include iron deposits at the base of the cone (Fleischer ring), bulging of the lower lid in downgaze (Munson sign – Fig. 109), central corneal oedema of sudden onset (acute hydrops – Fig. 109) and scarring.

Systemic associations   Include atopic dermatitis, osteogenesis imperfecta; syndromes – Down's, Turner's, Ehlers–Danlos, Marfan's.

Management
- Refractive correction with spectacles is initially adequate
- As progression occurs, correction with contact lenses
- Corneal grafting in advanced cases
- Supportive treatment for acute hydrops.

Keratoglobus

Very rare congenital bilateral thinning and protrusion of the entire cornea (Fig. 110). Acute hydrops may occur in some cases.

Megalocornea

Very rare, X-linked recessive condition with corneal diameters over 13 mm (Fig. 111). May develop lens subluxation.

Microcornea

Corneal diameters of less than 10 mm.

Classification
- *True microcornea*: globe of normal dimensions.
- *Sclerocornea*: 'scleralization' of the peripheral cornea makes it appear small
- *Microphthalmos*: small variably malformed globe (Fig. 112)
- *Nanophthalmos*: severe hypermetropia because of short axial length, but otherwise normal.

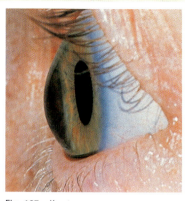

Fig. 107 Keratoconus.

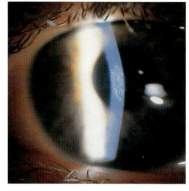

Fig. 108 Vogt's striae.

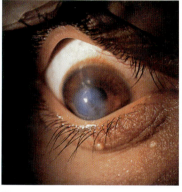

Fig. 109 Munson's sign in an eye with acute hydrops.

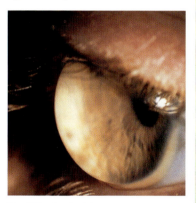

Fig. 110 Keratoglobus.

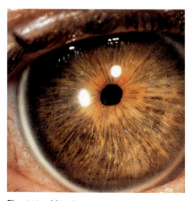

Fig. 111 Megalocornea.

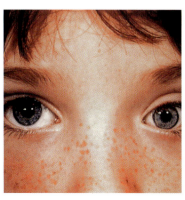

Fig. 112 Left microphthalmos.

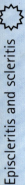

Episcleritis

Clinical features

This very common and innocuous condition presents with unilateral redness and slight discomfort.

Classification

- Nodular (Fig. 113)
- Diffuse (Fig. 114).

Management

Treatment is often not required. If necessary, topical steroids and systemic non-steroidal anti-inflammatory agents.

Scleritis

Deeper inflammation than episcleritis, with more severe symptoms and frequent systemic association.

Aetiology

Often idiopathic, but may follow eye surgery or be associated with herpes zoster or systemic disease such as rheumatoid arthritis, Wegener's granulomatosis and polyarteritis nodosa.

Classification

Anterior non-necrotizing   The most common type may be nodular (Fig. 115) or diffuse.

Anterior necrotizing with inflammation   Is a rare and painful condition characterized by local scleral injection and necrosis (Fig. 116). May be complicated by keratitis and anterior uveitis.

Scleromalacia perforans   Is rare and typically occurs in women with rheumatoid arthritis. It is characterized by uninflamed patches of scleral necrosis that expose the underlying uvea (Fig. 117). Spontaneous perforation is rare but may occur as a result of trauma. No benefit has been demonstrated from treatment.

Posterior scleritis

Clinical features

Uncommon and may be difficult to diagnose. Signs include proptosis, ophthalmoplegia, optic disc swelling, choroidal folds (see Fig. 40) and uveal effusion (Fig. 118).

Management

- Systemic non-steroidal anti-inflammatory agents
- Topical and/or systemic steroids
- Other immunosuppressive agents.

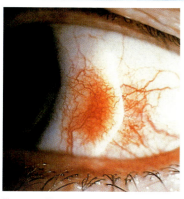

Fig. 113 Nodular episcleritis.

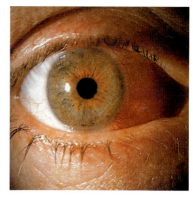

Fig. 114 Diffuse episcleritis.

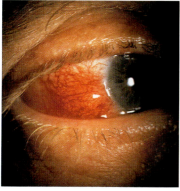

Fig. 115 Anterior non-necrotizing nodular scleritis.

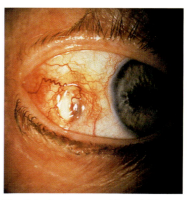

Fig. 116 Anterior necrotizing scleritis with inflammation.

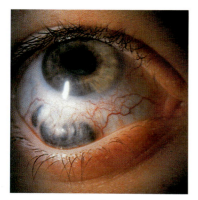

Fig. 117 Scleromalacia perforans.

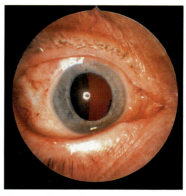

Fig. 118 Uveal effusion in scleritis.

Aetiology

Commonly idiopathic but numerous systemic associations/causes:

- *HLA-B27-associated*: ankylosing spondylitis, Reiter's syndrome, psoriatic arthritis
- *Juvenile idiopathic arthritis*: especially high-risk if pauciarticular-onset and ANA-positive
- *Inflammatory bowel disease*: ulcerative colitis, Crohn's disease
- *Non-infectious systemic diseases*: sarcoidosis, Behçet's disease, Vogt–Koyanagi–Harada syndrome
- *Infections*: herpes zoster and simplex, syphilis, tuberculosis
- *Idiopathic*: Fuchs' uveitis syndrome.

Clinical features

Symptoms

- *Acute iritis*: subacute onset of photophobia, redness, pain and blurred vision; usually unilateral
- *Chronic anterior uveitis*: symptoms may initially be absent or mild.

Signs

- *Acute iritis*: circumcorneal (ciliary) injection, small pupil, fine keratic precipitates ('KPs' – Figs 119, 120), aqueous flare (Fig. 120) and cells, white 'fluid level' (hypopyon – Fig. 121) and fibrinous exudate in severe inflammation
- *Chronic anterior uveitis*: usually little or no injection, KPs typically large ('mutton fat' in granulomatous inflammation, e.g. sarcoidosis), aqueous flare (Fig. 120) and cells (often fewer than in acute iritis), iris nodules (in granulomatous).

Complications

- Iris–lens adhesions (posterior synechiae – Fig. 122)
- Corneal calcium deposition (band keratopathy – Fig. 123)
- Cataract (Fig. 123)
- Glaucoma
- A blind, soft and shrunken globe (phthisis bulbi – Fig. 124) in end stage chronic uveitis.

Management

- Topical steroids and mydriatics are the mainstay of treatment
- Periocular steroid injection
- Systemic steroids, immunosuppressive agents and antibiotics for infections (e.g. tuberculosis, syphilis).

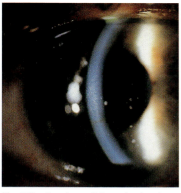

Fig. 119 Keratic precipitates in chronic anterior uveitis.

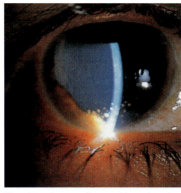

Fig. 120 Aqueous flare and large keratic precipitates.

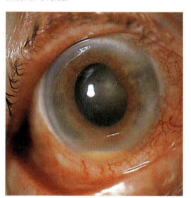

Fig. 121 Hypopyon in severe acute anterior uveitis.

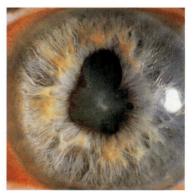

Fig. 122 Adhesions between the lens and iris (posterior synechiae).

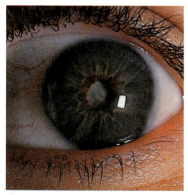

Fig. 123 Band keratopathy and cataract.

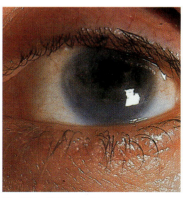

Fig. 124 Phthisis bulbi.

Toxoplasmosis

Aetiology
Reactivation of prenatal infection with the protozoan *Toxoplasma gondii.*

Clinical features
Subacute onset of unilateral vitreous floaters. Examination shows a moderate-severe vitritis associated with a solitary focus of retinitis adjacent to an old scar (Fig. 125).

Management
Treatment of vision-threatening lesions is with antimicrobial agents and systemic steroids. Special considerations apply to immunocompromised patients.

Toxocariasis

Aetiology
Rare infection caused by the common intestinal worm of dogs *Toxocara canis.*

Clinical features
- *Posterior pole granuloma*: presents with poor vision in one eye
- *Peripheral granuloma*: presents with distortion of the macula or disc (Fig. 126) or tractional retinal detachment (Fig. 127)
- *Chronic endophthalmitis*: presents with leukocoria (see Fig. 232), strabismus or visual loss.

Management
Vitrectomy may be considered for retinal detachment.

Cytomegalovirus (CMV) retinitis

Common in patients with AIDS, though less so with the introduction of newer drug regimens.

Clinical features
Yellow-white areas of retinal necrosis associated with variable haemorrhage and mild vitritis (Fig. 128). The lesions spread along the vascular arcades and may involve the optic nerve head (Fig. 129).

Management
Antiviral agents administered systemically, or intravitreally by injection or a slow-release implant.

Histoplasmosis

Aetiology
Infection with the fungus *Histoplasma capsulatum.*

Clinical features
Punched-out chorioretinal scars ('histo spots'), peripapillary atrophy (Fig. 130) and macular choroidal neovascularization (CNV); no associated vitritis.

Management
Laser photocoagulation or surgery may be appropriate for the CNV.

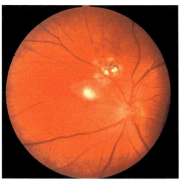

Fig. 125 Active retinal toxoplasmosis.

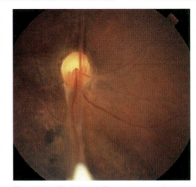

Fig. 126 Peripheral *Toxocara* granuloma.

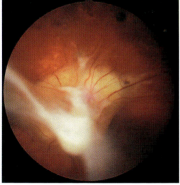

Fig. 127 Tractional retinal detachment in ocular toxocariasis.

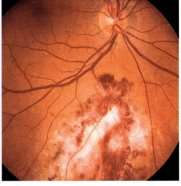

Fig. 128 Cytomegalovirus retinitis.

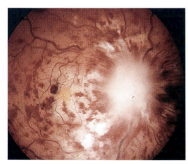

Fig. 129 Advanced cytomegalovirus retinitis with optic nerve involvement.

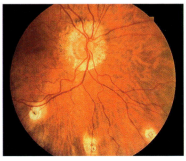

Fig. 130 Ocular histoplasmosis.

23 Non-infectious intermediate and posterior uveitis

Intermediate uveitis

Clinical features

Relatively common, often bilateral, chronic idiopathic inflammation of the pars plana (pars planitis) and retinal periphery of children and young adults, presenting with gradually increasing vitreous floaters. Examination shows vitritis (Fig. 131), often accompanied by exudate on the inferior pars plana ('snowbanking').

Complications

- Chronic cystoid macular oedema (main cause of severe visual loss)
- Cataract.

Management

Periocular depot steroid injection when visual acuity is reduced by cystoid macular oedema.

Sarcoidosis

Clinical features

Common idiopathic disease characterized by multisystem granulomatous inflammation. Anterior uveitis is common (see page 42); fundus signs include periphlebitis ('candlewax drippings' – Fig. 132), retinal, choroidal (Fig. 133) and optic nerve granulomata (Fig. 134), and peripheral retinal neovascularization.

Management

Systemic steroids.

Behçet's disease

Clinical features

Uncommon idiopathic multisystem disease characterized by aphthous oral ulceration, recurrent genital ulceration and skin lesions. Ocular features include periphlebitis, which may result in venous occlusion (Fig. 135), retinitis, macular oedema and optic atrophy (Fig. 136).

Management

Systemic steroids and immunosuppressive agents.

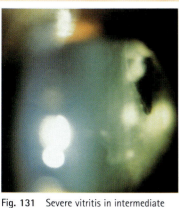

Fig. 131 Severe vitritis in intermediate uveitis.

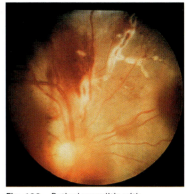

Fig. 132 Retinal vasculitis with 'candlewax' perivascular exudates.

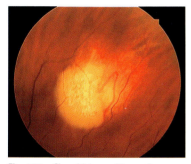

Fig. 133 Choroidal sarcoid granulomas.

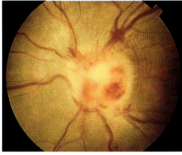

Fig. 134 Optic nerve head sarcoid granuloma.

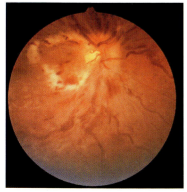

Fig. 135 Severe periphlebitis with venous occlusion in Behçet's disease.

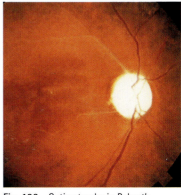

Fig. 136 Optic atrophy in Behçet's disease.

24 > Idiopathic multifocal white dot syndromes

'White dot syndromes' is the term for a heterogeneous group of rare inflammatory conditions of unknown aetiology which involve the posterior segment. Examples are presented below.

Birdshot retinochoroidopathy

Clinical features

Rare, idiopathic, chronic bilateral condition typically affecting middle-aged females who carry the genetic marker HLA-A29. Early lesions consist of multiple, deep, flat, creamy-yellow spots radiating outwards from the disc (Fig. 137), associated with variable vasculitis and vitritis. These evolve into circumscribed, atrophic white areas (Fig. 138). Cystoid macular oedema is very common; optic atrophy and cataract may also develop.

Management

Periocular and systemic steroids and immunosuppressive agents may be beneficial but the visual prognosis is guarded.

Acute multifocal posterior placoid pigment epitheliopathy (AMPPPE)

Clinical features

Uncommon, idiopathic, acute bilateral condition typically affecting young adults. Deep, oval, cream-coloured lesions (Fig. 139) develop initially, and on resolving leave variable pigmented scars (Fig. 140).

Management

The visual prognosis is usually excellent and no treatment is required.

Serpiginous choroidopathy

Clinical features

Rare, idiopathic, chronic bilateral condition of older patients. Cream-coloured lesions at the posterior pole (Fig. 141) evolve to leave atrophic areas (Fig. 142).

Management

Steroids and immunosuppressive agents may be tried but the visual prognosis is poor.

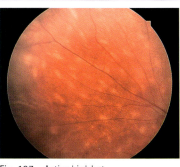

Fig. 137 Active birdshot retinochoroidopathy.

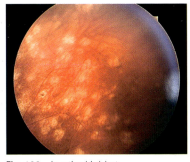

Fig. 138 Inactive birdshot retinochoroidopathy.

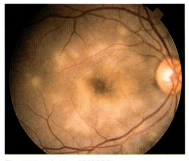

Fig. 139 Active AMPPPE.

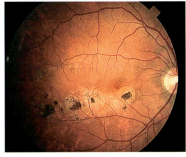

Fig. 140 Inactive AMPPPE.

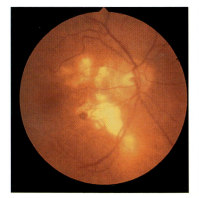

Fig. 141 Active serpiginous choroidopathy.

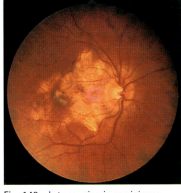

Fig. 142 Late scarring in serpiginous choroidopathy.

25 Primary open-angle glaucoma

Definition

Glaucoma is a progressive optic neuropathy in which the major risk factor for visual loss is elevated intraocular pressure (IOP – Fig. 143). In primary open-angle glaucoma (POAG), the most common of the glaucomas, raised IOP occurs secondarily to a gradual reduction in the drainage of aqueous humour via the trabecular meshwork. Glaucoma can be present, however, in the presence of normal IOP ('normal-tension' glaucoma).

Incidence

POAG affects at least 1% of the population over the age of 40 years. Both eyes are usually affected. The risk to siblings of affected individuals is approximately 10%.

Important risk factors

- High IOP
- Age
- Black race
- Family history
- Myopia.

Clinical features

Usually asymptomatic until significant loss of visual field has occurred. Frequently the condition is first suspected at a routine eye examination.

Signs

- Elevated IOP (>21 mmHg)
- Glaucomatous optic nerve damage (Figs 144–146)
- Visual field loss (Fig. 147)
- Open anterior chamber angle on gonioscopy.

Management

- Topical treatment (usually first-line) with beta-blockers, prostaglandin derivatives, carbonic anhydrase inhibitors, alpha-agonists and miotics
- Laser trabeculoplasty
- Filtration surgery, e.g. trabeculectomy (Fig. 148).

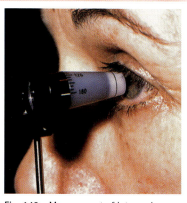

Fig. 143 Measurement of intraocular pressure.

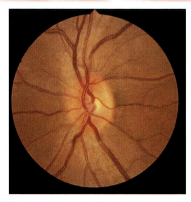

Fig. 144 Normal optic disc.

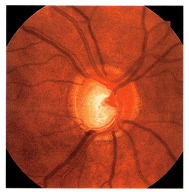

Fig. 145 Moderate cupping with inferior notching.

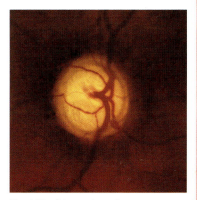

Fig. 146 Advanced cupping.

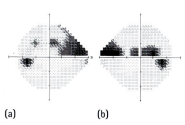

(a)   (b)

Fig. 147 Visual field loss in a glaucoma patient (a) left eye (b) right eye.

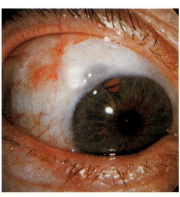

Fig. 148 Conjunctival filtration bleb following trabeculectomy.

26 > Secondary open-angle glaucomas

Pigmentary glaucoma

Aetiology

Blockage of aqueous outflow and secondary trabecular meshwork damage is caused by pigment granules derived from the iris.

Clinical features

Common: most patients are young myopic males.

Signs
- Vertical strip of pigment granules on the corneal endothelium (Krukenberg spindle – Fig. 149)
- Spoke-like transillumination defects in the mid-peripheral iris (Fig. 150)
- Gonioscopy: wide anterior chamber angle with heavily pigmented trabecular meshwork (Fig. 151)
- Other features: deep anterior chamber, pigment granules on the iris surface
- If no glaucomatous damage: 'pigment dispersion syndrome'.

Management

As for POAG.

Pseudoexfoliation glaucoma

Aetiology

Blockage of aqueous outflow by pseudoexfoliative material.

Clinical features

Common: typically affects the elderly.

Signs
- Pseudoexfoliative material on anterior lens surface (Fig. 152) and pupillary border (Fig. 153)
- Gonioscopy: trabecular hyperpigmentation and deposits of pseudoexfoliative material.

Management

As for POAG but may be more resistant to treatment.

Angle-recession glaucoma

Aetiology

Blunt traumatic trabecular damage.

Clinical features

Uncommon. Uniocular elevation of IOP, usually months or years after the initial injury. Examination clues to the diagnosis include signs of previous damage such as tears in the iris sphincter or iridodialysis (see Fig. 264), a slightly deeper anterior chamber than in the fellow eye, and a recessed and irregular angle on gonioscopy (Fig. 154).

Management

Treatment is initially medical although filtration surgery is often required eventually.

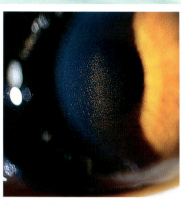

Fig. 149 Krukenberg spindle.

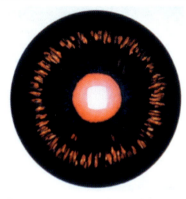

Fig. 150 Iris transillumination defects.

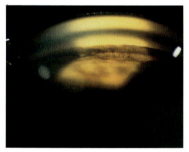

Fig. 151 Trabecular hyperpigmentation.

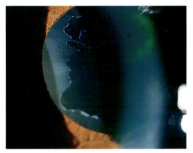

Fig. 152 Pseudoexfoliative material on the anterior lens capsule.

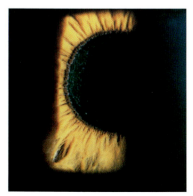

Fig. 153 Pseudoexfoliative material on the lens and pupil edge.

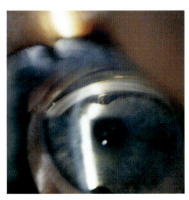

Fig. 154 Severe angle recession.

27 Primary angle–closure glaucoma

Definition

Elevation of IOP as a result of obstruction of the anterior chamber angle by the peripheral iris.

Aetiology

The normal increase in size of the lens with ageing may lead to narrowing of the anterior chamber angle. In an anatomically predisposed eye this can progress to obstruction.

Risk factors

- Increasing age (usually over 60)
- Female gender
- Hypermetropia, shallow anterior chamber and narrow angle.

Clinical features

Subacute angle-closure   Episodic transient blurring of vision and haloes around lights associated with aching and/or redness of the eye caused by intermittent angle closure that resolves spontaneously.

Chronic angle-closure   Gradual and insidious narrowing of the angle without acute symptoms, usually with gradual elevation of IOP.

Acute angle-closure   Sudden onset of total angle occlusion (Fig. 155) results in an acute and very severe increase in IOP with corresponding visual loss, ocular pain and redness, frequently accompanied by nausea and vomiting.

Signs of acute angle-closure glaucoma include:
- Very high IOP
- Circumcorneal (ciliary) injection
- Corneal oedema (Fig. 156)
- Fixed, mid-dilated, oval pupil (Fig. 157)
- Very shallow anterior chamber.

Signs following resolution of the acute attack:

- Iris atrophy (Fig. 158)
- Anterior lens opacity (*Glaukomflecken* – Fig. 159)

Management

- Treatment of acute glaucoma is with systemic carbonic anhydrase inhibitors, topical beta blockers, miotics alpha agonists and steroids; systemic osmotic agents may also be required
- Laser peripheral iridotomies (Fig. 160) once the cornea has cleared.

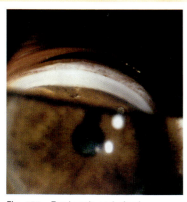

Fig. 155 Total angle occlusion by peripheral iris.

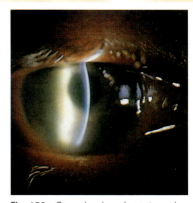

Fig. 156 Corneal oedema in acute angle-closure.

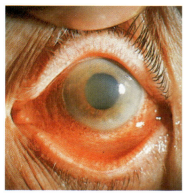

Fig. 157 Fixed mid-dilated pupil in acute angle-closure.

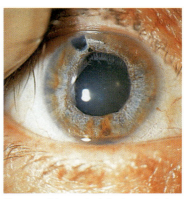

Fig. 158 Iris atrophy following resolution of acute angle-closure.

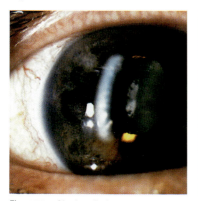

Fig. 159 *Glaukomflecken.*

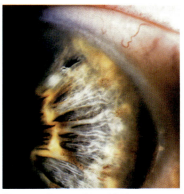

Fig. 160 Laser peripheral iridotomy.

28 Secondary angle-closure glaucomas

Neovascular glaucoma

Aetiology

Chronic retinal ischaemia leads to neovascularization on the iris (rubeosis iridis) and in the anterior chamber angle. Contraction of fibrovascular tissue (peripheral anterior synechiae – PAS) causes angle closure. Common causes are ischaemic central retinal vein occlusion (see Fig. 196), typically about 3 months after the thrombosis, and severe proliferative diabetic retinopathy.

Clinical features

Pain, decreased vision, anterior segment congestion, a very high IOP with corneal oedema, and severe rubeosis iridis (Figs 161, 162).

Management

- Panretinal photocoagulation if the fundus is visible, or peripheral retinal cryotherapy if not
- Topical atropine and steroids to decrease inflammation
- Filtration surgery (trabeculectomy with adjunctive antimetabolite, or drainage implant – Fig. 163)
- Partial ablation of the ciliary body with laser ('cyclodiode').

Inflammatory angle-closure glaucomas

Aetiology

Anterior uveitis may lead to angle-closure glaucoma via two mechanisms:

- 360° posterior synechiae (seclusio pupillae) causes iris bombé, a shallow anterior chamber and angle closure
- Without pupil block due to contraction of inflammatory debris in the angle with consequent PAS formation.

Iridocorneal endothelial (ICE) syndrome

Aetiology

Synechial angle closure by proliferation and contraction of abnormal corneal endothelial cells.

Clinical features

Rare. Typically affects one eye of a middle-aged woman. Signs include iris atrophy (Figs 165, 166), iris naevus or nodules and/or severe corneal endothelial changes.

Management

A drainage implant is often required.

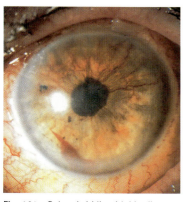

Fig. 161 Rubeosis iridis with bleeding from new vessels.

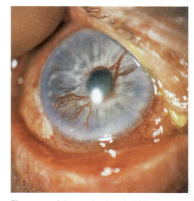

Fig. 162 Advanced rubeosis iridis.

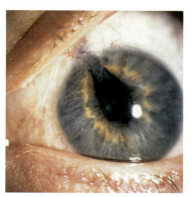

Fig. 163 Drainage implant.

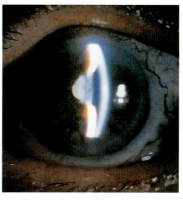

Fig. 164 Seclusio pupillae with shallow anterior chamber.

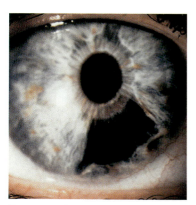

Fig. 165 Iris atrophy in ICE syndrome.

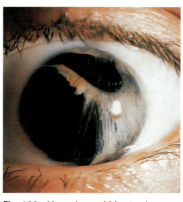

Fig. 166 Very advanced iris atrophy.

Primary congenital glaucoma

Incidence

1/10 000 live births; 65% are boys. Both eyes involved in 75% of cases, usually asymmetrically.

Clinical features

- Large eye (buphthalmos – Fig. 167) if IOP becomes elevated before age 3 years
- Breaks in Descemet's membrane (Haab striae – Fig. 168)
- Anterior chamber angle anomaly.

Management

- Incision of the trabecular meshwork (goniotomy)
- Less commonly trabeculotomy or trabeculectomy.

Iridocorneal dysgenesis

Definition

A spectrum of rare congenital disorders involving the anterior segment, sometimes associated with congenital or childhood glaucoma.

Classification

Axenfeld–Rieger syndrome   Posterior embryotoxon associated with extensive PAS, iris hypoplasia, holes, ectropion uveae and displaced pupil (Fig. 169).

Peters anomaly   Extremely rare condition characterized by a corneal scar associated with iris or lens adhesions (Fig. 170).

Aniridia   May be complete or partial (Fig. 171). Three phenotypes:

- *AN-1 (~66%)*: isolated ocular defect with autosomal dominant inheritance
- *AN-2 (~33%)*: sporadic; 30% chance of Wilms' tumour by age 5 years (Miller's syndrome)
- *AN-3 (1–2%)*: mental handicap and cerebellar ataxia (Gillespie's syndrome).

Phacomatoses

A group of conditions characterized by hamartomas in multiple organs. Congenital glaucoma may occur in:

- Sturge–Weber syndrome (Fig. 172); glaucoma in 30% of cases, due to either an angle anomaly or elevation of episcleral venous pressure.
- Neurofibromatosis-1; glaucoma is uncommon.

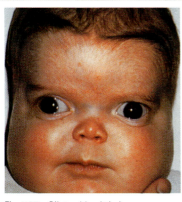

Fig. 167   Bilateral buphthalmos.

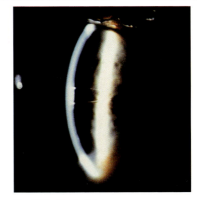

Fig. 168   Haab striae.

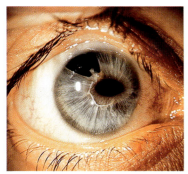

Fig. 169   Axenfeld–Rieger syndrome.

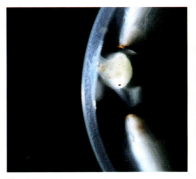

Fig. 170   Peters anomaly.

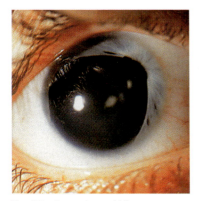

Fig. 171   Incomplete aniridia.

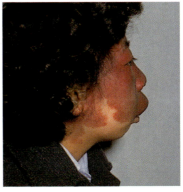

Fig. 172   Naevus flammeus in Sturge–Weber syndrome.

30 › Age-related cataract

Definition

Cataract is an opacity of the natural crystalline lens. It is an extremely common cause of visual impairment in older patients.

Classification

Subcapsular cataract May be anterior or posterior (Fig. 173). Patients experience glare and typically have more problems with reading than distance vision.

Nuclear cataract ('nuclear sclerosis') Consists of a central darkening of the lens (Fig. 174). It may cause an increase in myopia so that distance vision is affected more than near.

Cortical cataract – spoke-like opacities (Fig. 175).

Mature cataract – completely opaque lens with a white pupil (Fig. 176).

Management

Surgical extraction is the only treatment for cataract. The majority of modern cataract surgery is now carried out by means of phacoemulsification, in which the lens is removed through a narrow incision using a small-bore ultrasonic probe. The natural lens is replaced by an artificial intraocular lens implant (IOL – Fig. 177). Under special circumstances or where phacoemulsification equipment is not available, 'extracapsular' extraction is carried out, involving a larger corneal incision requiring sutures.

Complications

- Posterior lens capsular opacification (Fig. 178) occurs eventually in about 20% of cases; can be treated by YAG laser capsulotomy
- Acute or chronic bacterial endophthalmitis is rare but serious
- Expulsive (suprachoroidal) haemorrhage is a rare but potentially disastrous operative complication
- Retinal detachment is rare; myopes are particularly at risk.

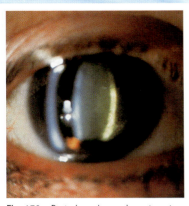

Fig. 173 Posterior subcapsular cataract.

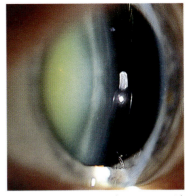

Fig. 174 Nuclear cataract (nuclear sclerosis).

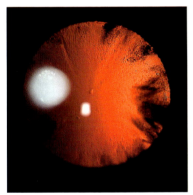

Fig. 175 Cortical cataract seen against the red reflex.

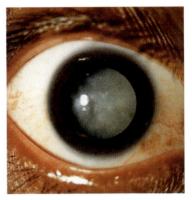

Fig. 176 Mature cataract.

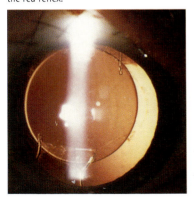

Fig. 177 Intraocular lens implant.

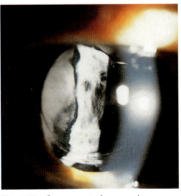

Fig. 178 Severe posterior capsular opacification.

Secondary cataract

Aetiology

- *Trauma*: penetrating, concussion, radiation and electric shock
- *Associated with ocular disease*: chronic anterior uveitis (see Fig. 123), high myopia, acute angle-closure glaucoma (see Fig. 159), hereditary retinal dystrophies
- *Associated with systemic disease*: diabetes, myotonic dystrophy atopic dermatitis
- *Drug-induced*: most commonly systemic steroids.

Infantile cataract

Aetiology

- *Idiopathic sporadic*: may be unilateral
- *Hereditary*: most frequently autosomal dominant
- *Associated with other ocular malformations*: persistent hyperplastic primary vitreous, retinopathy of prematurity, aniridia (see Fig. 171), Peters anomaly (see Fig. 170)
- *Embryopathies*: intrauterine infections (e.g. rubella, toxoplasmosis)
- *Metabolic*: galactokinase deficiency, galactosaemia and hypocalcaemia
- *Syndromes*: Lowe, Down, Turner and *cri du chat*.

Clinical features

Appearance of infantile cataract is variable (Figs 179, 180).

Ectopia lentis

Definition

Displacement of the lens; may be partial (subluxation) or complete.

Aetiology

- *Trauma* (Fig. 181)
- *Familial ectopia lentis*: may be associated with ectopic pupil (Fig. 182)
- *Associated with other ocular disorders*: aniridia (see Fig. 171) and buphthalmos (see Fig. 167)
- *Syndromes*: Marfan's (Fig. 183) and Weill–Marchesani
- *Metabolic*: homocystinuria and hyperlysinaemia.

Abnormalities of lens size and shape

- *Microphakia*: small lens
- *Microspherophakia*: small spherical lens
- *Coloboma*: (Fig. 184) may be associated with colobomas of the iris and choroid, and giant retinal tears
- *Lenticonus*: cone-shaped lens surface (e.g. anterior lenticonus in Alport syndrome).

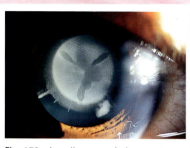

Fig. 179   Lamellar congenital cataract.

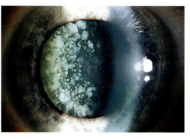

Fig. 180   Punctate congenital lens opacities.

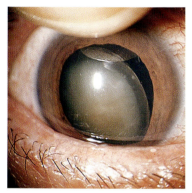

Fig. 181   Lens subluxation due to blunt trauma.

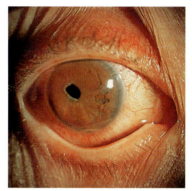

Fig. 182   Congenital ectopic pupil with associated lens subluxation.

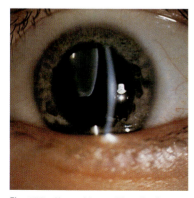

Fig. 183   Upward lens subluxation in Marfan's syndrome.

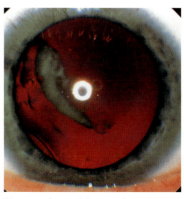

Fig. 184   Lens coloboma and opacity.

Incidence

Diabetic retinopathy (DR) is the most common cause of blindness in the working-age population. The incidence and severity of DR are strongly related to duration of diabetes; good control of blood glucose and hypertension are very important.

Clinical features

Background DR   Microaneurysms, dot and blot haemorrhages and hard exudates (Figs 185, 186).

Preproliferative DR   Cotton-wool spots, intraretinal microvascular anomalies (IRMA), venous changes (beading, looping and segmentation) and dark blot haemorrhages (Fig. 187).

Proliferative diabetic retinopathy   New vessel formation at the optic disc (NVD – Fig. 188) or elsewhere on the retina (NVE – Fig. 189). Severe visual loss may occur as a result of vitreous haemorrhage or tractional retinal detachment due to contraction of fibrovascular tissue (see Fig. 224).

Diabetic maculopathy   Maculopathy is the most common cause of visual impairment in patients with diabetes. Loss of visual function is usually caused by oedema, typically accompanied by exudates. Less commonly, the macula becomes ischaemic, often with severe deterioration in central vision.

Management

- Regular review if treatment is not indicated, frequency dependent on severity of DR
- Panretinal laser photocoagulation for proliferative DR (Fig. 190)
- Grid or focal laser photocoagulation for macular oedema fitting certain criteria ('clinically significant macular oedema')
- Vitrectomy for persistent vitreous haemorrhage or tractional retinal detachment involving the centre of the macula.

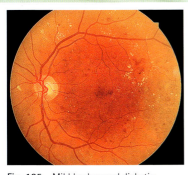

Fig. 185 Mild background diabetic retinopathy.

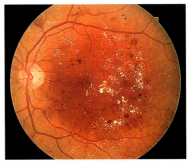

Fig. 186 Severe background diabetic retinopathy.

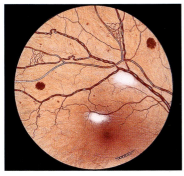

Fig. 187 Pre-proliferative diabetic retinopathy.

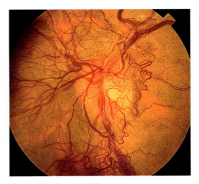

Fig. 188 Severe NVD.

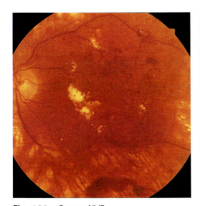

Fig. 189 Severe NVE.

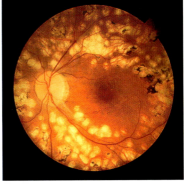

Fig. 190 Laser scars following panretinal photocoagulation.

Retinal vein occlusion (RVO)

Aetiology

Predisposing factors include increasing age, hypertension, hyperviscosity, vasculitis, thrombophilic disorders and raised IOP.

Clinical features

Presents with sudden mild to severe loss of vision in one eye. Acute signs include haemorrhages, cotton wool spots, venous tortuosity, optic disc and retinal oedema.

Classification

- *Branch RVO* (Fig. 191): usually involves a retinal quadrant
- *Hemiretinal vein occlusion* (Fig. 192)
- *Central RVO*: ischaemic or non-ischaemic (Fig. 193).

Complications

- Retinal neovascularization, especially in BRVO, is treated with laser photocoagulation
- Macular oedema is treated with grid laser photocoagulation to the macula in selected cases
- Neovascular glaucoma (see Fig. 161) in ischaemic CRVO.

Retinal artery occlusion (RAO)

Aetiology

Embolization from a carotid or cardiac source, or vaso-obliteration by atheroma or arteritis.

Clinical features

Acute loss of vision; may be permanent or transient (amaurosis fugax). Retinal pallor corresponding to the involved area (central or branch) is seen (Fig. 194), and in central RAO a 'cherry red spot' at the fovea is typically present (Fig. 195). Segmentation of the arteriolar blood column ('cattle trucking') may be seen. Later the arterioles become attenuated and the optic disc pale.

Management

- Urgent erythrocyte sedimentation rate (ESR) to exclude giant cell arteritis and investigation of other risk factors
- Amaurosis fugax: aspirin; carotid endarterectomy for severe stenosis
- Acute RAO may be relieved by lowering IOP by massage, intravenous acetazolamide, anterior chamber paracentesis.

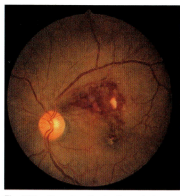

Fig. 191 Branch retinal vein occlusion.

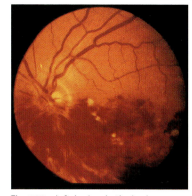

Fig. 192 Inferior hemiretinal vein occlusion.

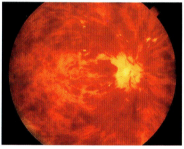

Fig. 193 Central retinal vein occlusion.

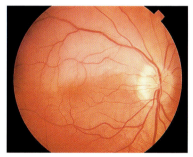

Fig. 194 Branch retinal artery occlusion.

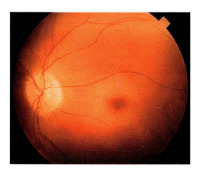

Fig. 195 Central retinal artery occlusion with 'cherry-red spot'.

34 > Miscellaneous retinopathies

Hypertensive retinopathy

Classification
- *Grade 1*: mild generalized arteriolar narrowing (Fig. 196)
- *Grade 2*: focal as well as marked generalized arteriolar constriction (Fig. 197)
- *Grade 3*: as Grade 2 plus retinal haemorrhages, cotton wool spots and hard exudates (Fig. 198)
- *Grade 4*: as Grade 3 plus optic disc swelling (Fig. 199).

Sickle-cell retinopathy

Patients typically have SC or SThal disease.

Classification
- *Stage 1*: peripheral arteriolar occlusion
- *Stage 2*: peripheral arteriovenous anastomoses
- *Stage 3*: growth of extraretinal new vessels from anastomoses
- *Stage 4*: vitreous haemorrhage (Fig. 200)
- *Stage 5*: tractional retinal detachment.

Management
A high rate of spontaneous infarction of ischaemic areas means that photocoagulation is rarely performed but vitrectomy may be required for stage 4 and 5 disease.

Retinopathy of prematurity (ROP)

Definition
Proliferative retinopathy affecting low-birth-weight preterm infants exposed to high ambient levels of oxygen.

Classification
- *Stage 1*: demarcation mark parallel to the ora serrata
- *Stage 2*: ridge with associated neovascular tufts
- *Stage 3*: fibrovascular proliferation from the ridge (Fig. 201)
- *Stage 4*: subtotal tractional retinal detachment
- *Stage 5*: total retinal detachment
- *'Plus' disease*: vitreous haze, posterior pole vascular tortuosity
- *Cicatricial ROP*: complications due to fibrosis following involution of acute disease.

Management
- Structured screening of at-risk infants
- Treatment with peripheral retinal cryotherapy or laser photocoagulation for 'threshold' disease.

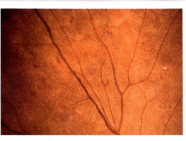

Fig. 196 Generalized arteriolar constriction in Grade 1 hypertensive retinopathy.

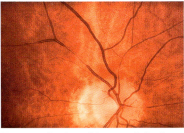

Fig. 197 Focal arteriolar constriction in Grade 2 hypertensive retinopathy.

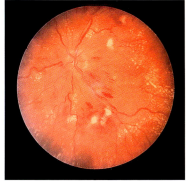

Fig. 198 Haemorrhages, cotton wool spots and hard exudates in Grade 3 hypertensive retinopathy.

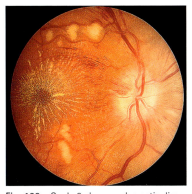

Fig. 199 Grade 3 changes plus optic disc swelling and a macular star in Grade 4 hypertensive retinopathy.

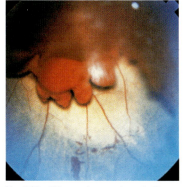

Fig. 200 Vitreous haemorrhage in Stage 4 sickle-cell retinopathy.

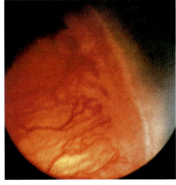

Fig. 201 Ridge with fibrovascular proliferation in Stage 3 ROP.

Incidence

Age-related macular degeneration (AMD) is the most common cause of legal blindness in industrialized societies. Patients are typically over the age of 65 years; both eyes are usually affected, frequently asymmetrically.

Clinical features

Hard drusen   Small, round, discrete, yellow-white lesions, usually located at the macula (Fig. 202).

Soft drusen   Larger lesions with ill-defined edges (Fig. 203) associated with exudative AMD.

Non-exudative ('dry') macular degeneration   Atrophic and hyperplastic changes of the retinal pigment epithelium (RPE) associated with slowly progressive degeneration of the overlying neuroretina and underlying choriocapillaris (Fig. 204).

Exudative ('wet') macular degeneration   The ingrowth of choroidal new vessels through Bruch membrane: choroidal neovascularization (CNV). Presents with unilateral distortion of central vision. On examination, an area of the macula is elevated by subretinal fluid or blood (Fig. 205), often with associated clumps of exudates (Fig. 206). The lesion evolves in most cases to leave subretinal 'disciform' scarring with permanent loss of central vision (Fig. 207).

RPE detachment (PED)   Fluid elevates the RPE in a dome configuration. This may progress to exudative AMD described above or may occasionally settle spontaneously.

Polypoidal choroidal vasculopathy (PCV)   This recently-described form of AMD may masquerade as CNV. Its behaviour, particularly the response to treatment, has yet to be clearly defined.

Management

- Often of negligible or temporary benefit and therefore only used in selected cases
- Antioxidant vitamin and mineral supplements may retard the progression of AMD
- Conventional laser may be effective at destroying CNV that does not encroach on the central macula
- Photodynamic therapy (PDT) is a newer technique using a laser to activate a light-sensitive dye preferentially taken up by CNV.

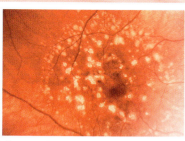

Fig. 202 Macular hard drusen.

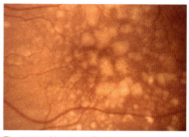

Fig. 203 Macular soft drusen.

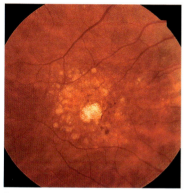

Fig. 204 Early 'dry' macular degeneration.

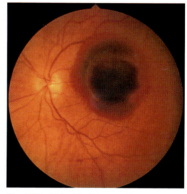

Fig. 205 Subretinal haemorrhage associated with CNV.

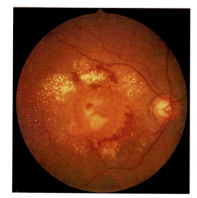

Fig. 206 Intra- and subretinal exudation associated with CNV.

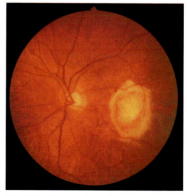

Fig. 207 Advanced disciform scarring.

Macular hole

The visual deficit is often noticed by chance when one eye is closed. On examination a rounded punched-out area measuring one-third of a disc diameter is seen at the fovea, surrounded by a grey halo of retinal elevation (Fig. 208). Treatment in early cases is by vitrectomy and intraocular gas.

Myopic maculopathy

Presentation of this common disorder is with either unilateral metamorphopsia or impaired visual acuity. On examination, a variety of changes may be seen: pigment proliferation (Fuchs spot – Fig. 209), atrophic maculopathy (Fig. 210), breaks in the Bruch membrane ('lacquer cracks') and macular haemorrhage.

Macular epiretinal membrane

This proliferation of glial cells and associated fibrous tissue across the retinal surface is often idiopathic but may occur following retinal disease, surgery or trauma. Presentation is with unilateral distortion and blurring of gradual onset. An early membrane may be subtle ('cellophane maculopathy') and manifest mild retinal wrinkling and vascular tortuosity. As a membrane thickens and contracts, the changes become more evident ('macular pucker' – Fig. 211).

Angioid streaks

In this rare binocular condition, linear streaks are seen radiating from the optic disc (Fig. 212). Vision can be affected, particularly by CNV. About 50% of individuals with angioid streaks have pseudoxanthoma elasticum.

Bull's eye maculopathy

Central foveolar hyperpigmentation surrounded by a depigmented zone encircled in turn by a hyperpigmented ring (Fig. 213). Causes include antimalarial drugs, cone dystrophy, Stargardt disease (see Fig. 215) and Batten disease.

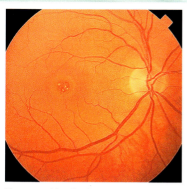

Fig. 208   Macular hole.

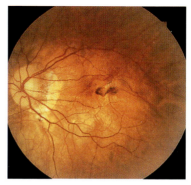

Fig. 209   Myopic maculopathy: Fuchs spot

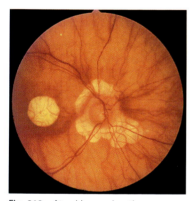

Fig. 210   Atrophic maculopathy.

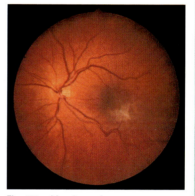

Fig. 211   Macular pucker.

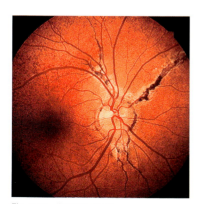

Fig. 212   Angioid streaks.

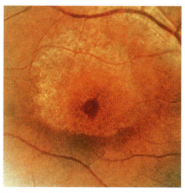

Fig. 213   Bull's eye maculopathy.

37 Dystrophies of the fundus

Retinitis pigmentosa

Presentation of this uncommon condition is during the second decade of life with night blindness. Inheritance may be autosomal dominant, recessive or X-linked. A large number of genetic abnormalities have been found to cause the clinical picture, the hallmarks of which are mid-peripheral perivascular 'bone-spicule' pigmentation, arteriolar attenuation and waxy disc pallor (Fig. 214). Associated macular oedema and cataract are common. A number of systemic syndromes are associated.

Stargardt's disease and fundus flavimaculatus

These two uncommon conditions represent variants of the same underlying autosomal recessive disease. Presentation is with central visual impairment: in early adulthood in Stargardt's and early middle age in fundus flavimaculatus. In early Stargardt's disease a 'beaten-bronze' macular lesion is seen that slowly progresses to an atrophic lesion (Fig. 215). In fundus flavimaculatus yellow-white flecks are scattered throughout the posterior pole and mid-peripheral fundus (Fig. 216), and maculopathy similar to Stargardt's may develop.

Best's disease

In this rare dominantly inherited disorder the macular appearance evolves over time from a juvenile egg yolk (vitelliform) lesion (Fig. 217) to scarring and severe visual loss in adult life.

Choroidal dystrophies

Choroideremia   Very rare X-linked disorder presenting during the first decade with night blindness characterized by enlarging midretinal patches of chorioretinal atrophy that progressively spread centrally but spare the macula till late on (Fig. 218).

Gyrate atrophy   Very rare recessively inherited inborn error of metabolism presenting during the first decade with night blindness characterized by coalescing midretinal patches of chorioretinal atrophy (Fig. 219).

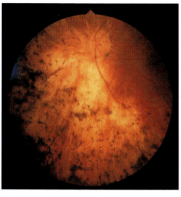

Fig. 214   Retinitis pigmentosa.

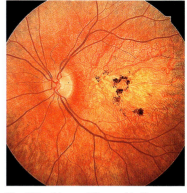

Fig. 215   Advanced Stargardt's disease.

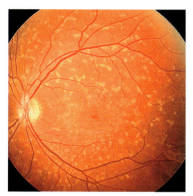

Fig. 216   Fundus flavimaculatus.

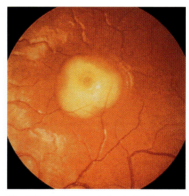

Fig. 217   Vitelliform lesion in Best's disease.

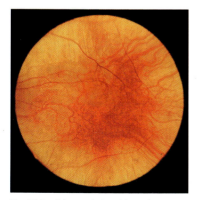

Fig. 218   Advanced choroideremia.

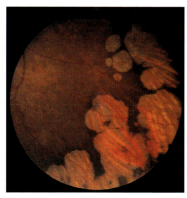

Fig. 219   Gyrate atrophy.

38 Retinal detachment

Definition	A separation of the neuroretina from the underlying retinal pigment epithelium (RPE) by the accumulation of subretinal fluid (SRF).

Rhegmatogenous retinal detachment

Aetiology	A retinal tear (Fig. 220) develops as a result of vitreoretinal traction on a weak area in the peripheral retina (e.g. lattice degeneration – Fig. 221).
Clinical features	• *Acute*: mobile convex, slightly opaque, corrugated detached retina (Fig. 222) with break(s) • *Long-standing*: retinal thinning, cysts, demarcation lines ('high water marks'), and fibrotic and immobile retina (proliferative vitreoretinopathy – PVR – Fig. 223).
Management	• Scleral buckling for uncomplicated cases • Vitrectomy combined with intravitreal injection of gas or silicone oil for complicated cases.

Tractional retinal detachment

Contraction of fibrous tissue, e.g. associated with proliferative diabetic retinopathy, causes the retina to detach without a break; on examination concave immobile retina with shallow SRF is seen (Fig. 224). Treated by pars plana vitrectomy.

Exudative retinal detachment

Aetiology	The passage of fluid from the choroid into the subretinal space occurs following breakdown of physiological barriers. Causes include intraocular tumours, inflammation, severe CNV, extensive laser photocoagulation and severe hypertension.
Clinical features	Convex, very mobile retina with deep shifting fluid and absence of retinal breaks (Fig. 225). Treatment consists of addressing the cause.

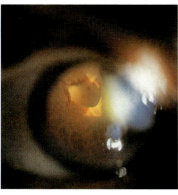

Fig. 220 Large retinal tear.

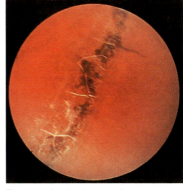

Fig. 221 Lattice degeneration.

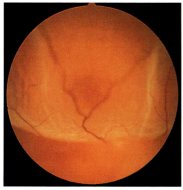

Fig. 222 Acute superior rhegmatogenous retinal detachment.

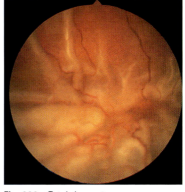

Fig. 223 Total rhegmatogenous detachment with severe PVR.

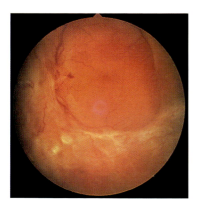

Fig. 224 Tractional retinal detachment.

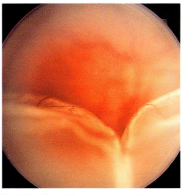

Fig. 225 Exudative retinal detachment.

39 | Tumours of the uvea

Choroidal naevus

Clinical features

This common benign tumour is a flat or slightly elevated, oval or round, slate-grey lesion, usually less than 3 mm in diameter. Overlying drusen are often present (Fig. 226).

Choroidal melanoma

Clinical features

This is the most common primary malignant intraocular tumour in adults. Examination shows a pigmented or amelanotic subretinal mass associated with exudative retinal detachment (Fig. 227)

Management

Options include enucleation, plaque or external beam irradiation, laser photocoagulation or local resection.

Iris melanoma

Clinical features

A pigmented or non-pigmented inferior iris nodule (Fig. 228) which may be associated with pupillary distortion, ectropion uveae and iris neovascularization.

Choroidal haemangioma

Clinical features

A very rare dome-shaped or placoid, orange-red lesion typically located at the posterior pole (Fig. 229) which may be associated with secondary cystoid degeneration and pigment mottling.

Metastatic carcinoma

Clinical features

Solitary or multiple, unilateral or bilateral, creamy-white, oval lesions with ill-defined borders, most commonly located at the posterior pole (Fig. 230). Common primary sites are the bronchus and breast.

Choroidal osteoma

Clinical features

This very rare tumour typically presents in a young female as a slightly elevated, orange-yellow lesion with well-demarcated borders, located at the posterior pole (Fig. 231). 25% are eventually bilateral.

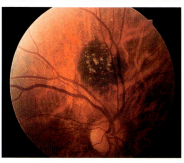

Fig. 226 Choroidal naevus with overlying drusen.

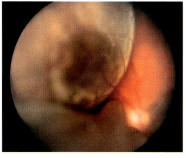

Fig. 227 Large choroidal melanoma with exudative retinal detachment.

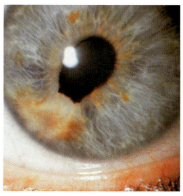

Fig. 228 Iris melanoma.

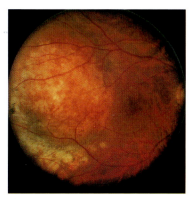

Fig. 229 Choroidal haemangioma with exudative retinal detachment.

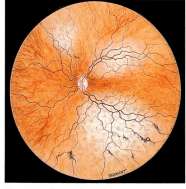

Fig. 230 Three choroidal metastases.

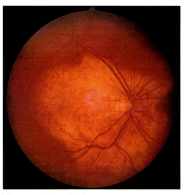

Fig. 231 Choroidal osteoma.

40 Tumours of the retina and optic nerve head

Retinoblastoma

Clinical features

The most common malignant ocular tumour in children. Bilateral in 30% of cases; 6% of patients have a positive family history. Presents typically at about 18 months with a white pupil (leukocoria – Fig. 232) and grows either into the vitreous cavity (endophytic) or in the subretinal space (exophytic).

Management

Options include external beam or plaque irradiation, laser photocoagulation, cryotherapy, systemic chemotherapy, and enucleation.

Retinal astrocytoma

Clinical features

An uncommon, benign tumour that typically affects patients with tuberous sclerosis (Bourneville's disease). Whitish, round mass frequently situated near the optic nerve head (Fig. 233). May be multiple and bilateral.

Retinal capillary haemangioma

Clinical features

Uncommon benign tumour. Round, orange-red lesion associated with dilated supplying and draining vessels (Fig. 234). Frequently multiple, with both eyes affected in 50% of cases. 25% of patients have systemic lesions (von Hippel–Lindau syndrome). Treatment involves laser photocoagulation or cryotherapy.

Retinal cavernous haemangioma

Very rare congenital lesion characterized by grape-like aneurysmal clusters (Fig. 235).

Retinal racemose haemangioma

A very rare congenital arteriovenous malformation consisting of grossly dilated and tortuous vessels (Fig. 236). A proportion of patients will have central nervous system lesions (Wyburn–Mason syndrome).

Melanocytoma of the optic nerve head

Rare, benign black tumour with feathery edges (Fig. 237) which usually occurs in pigmented races.

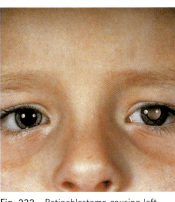

Fig. 232 Retinoblastoma causing left leukocoria.

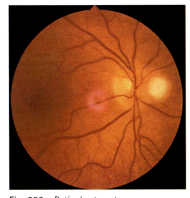

Fig. 233 Retinal astrocytoma.

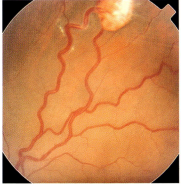

Fig. 234 Retinal capillary haemangioma.

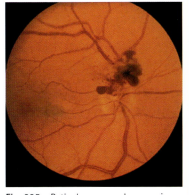

Fig. 235 Retinal cavernous haemangioma.

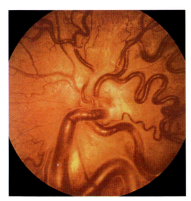

Fig. 236 Retinal racemose haemangioma.

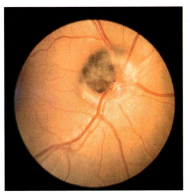

Fig. 237 Melanocytoma of the optic nerve head.

Optic neuritis

Definition

Inflammation of the optic nerve, with a range of causes, the most important being multiple sclerosis.

Clinical features

Presents with subacute, usually unilateral, impairment of central vision that may be associated with pain, especially on eye movement. The optic disc is usually normal (retrobulbar neuritis) and occasionally swollen (papillitis). Severe or recurrent attacks may lead to optic atrophy (Fig. 238).

Anterior ischaemic optic neuropathy

Definition

Infarction of the optic nerve head.

Classification

- *Arteritic*: associated with giant cell arteritis and has a poor prognosis
- *Non-arteritic*: associated with hypertension and atherosclerosis.

Clinical features

Presents with severe acute unilateral visual loss (arteritic) or variable visual decrease associated with an altitudinal visual field defect (non-arteritic). On examination, the optic disc is pale and swollen. Splinter-shaped haemorrhages are common (Fig. 239).

Management

An immediate ESR is essential. The arteritic form is treated with high-dose systemic steroids to protect the other eye.

Papilloedema

Definition

Disc swelling caused by raised intracranial pressure.

Clinical features

Symptoms of raised intracranial pressure including headaches and nausea. Transient visual obscuration lasting a few seconds are common but visual acuity is normal until late.

Signs

- *Early*: hyperaemia with indistinct margins (Fig. 240)
- *Established*: obvious elevation, peripapillary haemorrhages (Fig. 241) and cotton wool spots
- *Long-standing*: markedly elevated 'champagne cork' appearance (Fig. 242).

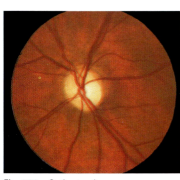

Fig. 238 Optic atrophy.

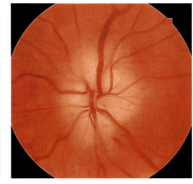

Fig. 239 Anterior ischaemic optic neuropathy.

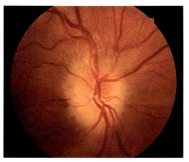

Fig. 240 Early papilloedema.

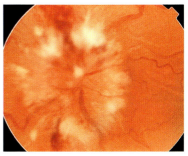

Fig. 241 Established papilloedema.

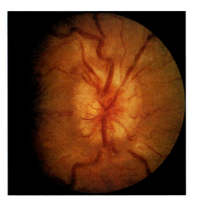

Fig. 242 Long-standing papilloedema.

Clinical features

Tilted disc

Oval optic disc with its vertical axis directed obliquely (Fig. 243) often associated with myopia and usually bilateral. A stable upper temporal visual field defect that fails to respect the vertical midline is frequent.

Optic disc drusen

Deposits of hyaline-like material within the optic nerve head which are often bilateral and familial.

May mimic the appearance of optic disc swelling (pseudopapilloedema). The optic nerve head is lumpy and elevated, with no physiological cup. Emerging blood vessels branch anomalously (Fig. 244). Visual field defects or choroidal neovascularisation may occur.

Myelinated nerve fibres

Persistent myelination of the retinal nerve fibres. Feathery white patches which may be mistaken for papilloedema when located around the optic disc (Fig. 245).

Optic disc pit

Usually unilateral dark, round or oval pit in a larger than normal disc (Fig. 246). About 50% of eyes develop a serous detachment of the macula.

Optic disc coloboma

Caused by defective closure of the fetal fissure. The optic nerve head contains a large inferior excavation (Fig. 247). Visual acuity is usually impaired and a superior visual field defect is typical. May be associated with a variety of congenital neurological and systemic anomalies.

Morning glory anomaly

The disc is enlarged and excavated with hyaloid remnants within its base and blood vessels emerging radially (Fig. 248). Vision may be severely impaired. Associated congenital central nervous system and other midline defects may be present.

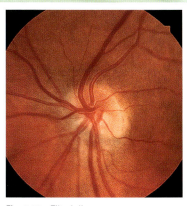

Fig. 243   Tilted disc.

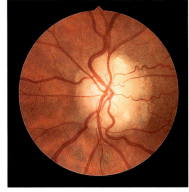

Fig. 244   Optic disc drusen.

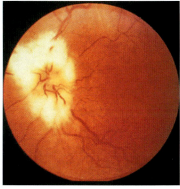

Fig. 245   Myelinated nerve fibres.

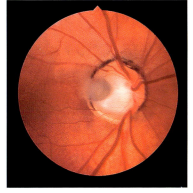

Fig. 246   Optic disc pit.

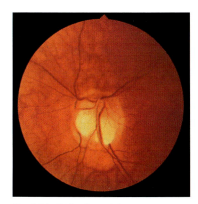

Fig. 247   Optic disc coloboma.

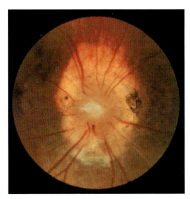

Fig. 248   Morning glory anomaly.

Strabismus

Definition

A misalignment of the eyes.

Esotropia (convergent squint)

Clinical features

Infantile esotropia   Presentation is in the first 6 months of life; should not be confused with pseudoesotropia (Fig. 249). Constant large angle (Fig. 250), occasionally inferior oblique overaction and nystagmus.

Accommodative esotropia   Convergent squint linked with focussing, typically presenting at about 2.5 years. In some cases, the eyes can be straightened by spectacle correction of a hypermetropic refractive error.

Non-accommodative esotropia   Includes sensory esotropia, caused by loss of vision in one eye impairing fusion, and consecutive esotropia, occurring after surgery to correct exotropia.

Exotropia (divergent squint– Fig. 251)

Classification

- *Congenital*
- *Intermittent*: in infants and older children
- *Secondary*: similar to esotropic counterpart
- *Consecutive*: following surgery for esotropia.

Duane's syndrome

Clinical features

Uncommon congenital condition, bilateral in 20% of cases. Eyes are usually straight in the primary position but abduction severely restricted (Fig. 252), with retraction of the globe and narrowing of the palpebral fissure on adduction (Fig. 253).

Brown's syndrome

Clinical features

Rare congenital condition, bilateral in 10% of cases. Eyes straight in the primary position, but there is limited elevation in adduction (Fig. 254).

Management of squint

- Ophthalmoscopy to exclude media opacity or fundus lesion
- Correction of significant refractive error
- Treatment of amblyopia (usually occlusion therapy)
- Extraocular muscle surgery, if appropriate.

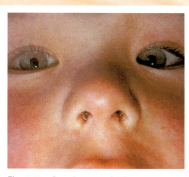

Fig. 249 Pseudoesotropia due to epicanthic folds. Note symmetrical corneal reflexes.

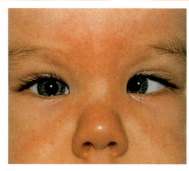

Fig. 250 Left infantile esotropia. Note asymmetrical corneal reflexes.

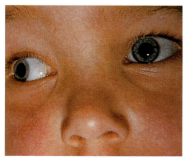

Fig. 251 Right exotropia.

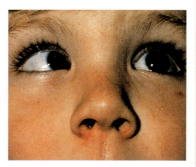

Fig. 252 Left Duane's syndrome; attempted abduction of the left eye.

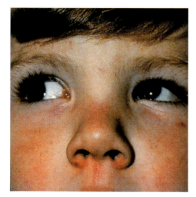

Fig. 253 Left Duane's syndrome; note retraction of the left eye on adduction.

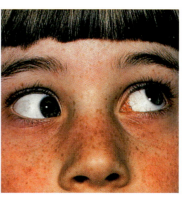

Fig. 254 Right Brown's syndrome.

44 > Third, fourth and sixth nerve palsies

Clinical features

Third (oculomotor) nerve palsy

- Ptosis due to paralysis of the levator palpebrae superioris
- Divergence due to unopposed action of the lateral rectus
- Defective elevation due to paralysis of the superior rectus and inferior oblique muscles (Fig. 255)
- Defective depression due to paralysis of the inferior rectus (Fig. 256)
- Defective adduction due to paralysis of the medial rectus (Fig. 257)
- Intorsion on attempted downgaze (unopposed superior oblique)
- Internal ophthalmoplegia – dilated, poorly reactive pupil and defective accommodation.

Fourth (trochlear) nerve palsy

- Hyperdeviation (latent or manifest) in the primary position; accentuated by ipsilateral head tilt: positive Bielschowsky test (Fig. 258)
- Defective depression in adduction (Fig. 259)
- Vertical diplopia, worse in downgaze

Sixth (abducens) nerve palsy

- Horizontal diplopia most marked in abduction
- Convergence in the primary position due to unopposed medial rectus
- Limitation of abduction (Fig. 260).

Aetiology

- *Vascular disease* (e.g. atherosclerosis, hypertension, diabetes): isolated or as part of larger stroke
- *Posterior communicating artery aneurysm*: consider in 3rd nerve palsy especially if painful, pupil involved and absence of vascular risk factors
- *Raised intracranial pressure*: bilateral 6th nerve palsy (false localizing sign)
- *Trauma*: especially bilateral 4th nerve palsy
- *Cavernous sinus lesions* (e.g. fistula, thrombosis): 4th and 6th nerve palsy
- *Tumours* (e.g. acoustic neuroma, nasopharyngeal carcinoma): 6th nerve palsy.

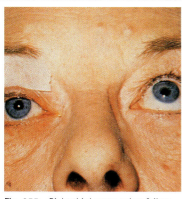

Fig. 255 Right third nerve palsy: failure of elevation.

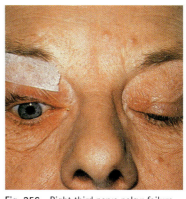

Fig. 256 Right third nerve palsy: failure of depression.

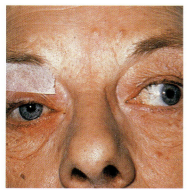

Fig. 257 Right third nerve palsy: failure of adduction.

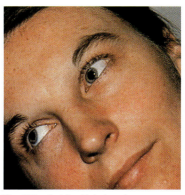

Fig. 258 Positive Bielschowsky test showing right hyperdeviation.

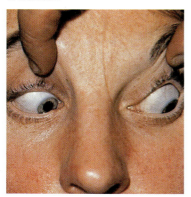

Fig. 259 Right fourth nerve palsy: failure of depression in adduction.

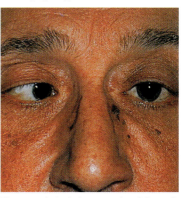

Fig. 260 Left sixth nerve palsy: failure of abduction.

45 Trauma

Corneal abrasion

Clinical features

Very common and often caused by fingernails and plant stems. Pain is marked and associated with blepharospasm and lacrimation. The epithelial defect, which stains with fluorescein (Fig. 261), often heals within 24 hours. Some patients subsequently develop recurrent corneal erosions.

Management

Antibiotic ointment; padding may improve comfort in very large abrasions but does not enhance healing.

Foreign body

Clinical features

- *Subtarsal*: usually scratches the superior cornea with blinking
- *Corneal foreign body*: typically ferrous and may be associated with a surrounding rust ring (Fig. 262)
- *Penetrating*: commonly hammered metal fragments. Complications include infection and cataract.

Blunt anterior segment trauma

- *Subconjunctival haemorrhage and periocular ecchymosis*
- *Hyphaema* (Fig. 263): re-bleeding may result in a severe IOP rise with a risk of corneal blood staining
- *Iris sphincter damage*
- *Iridodialysis* (Fig. 264)
- *Angle recession* (see Fig. 154): risk of chronic glaucoma
- *Lens damage*: subluxation, dislocation (see Fig. 181) and cataract formation
- *Scleral rupture:* usually caused by severe trauma.

Blunt posterior segment trauma

- *Vitreous haemorrhage*: may hide underlying damage; ultrasound indicated
- *Commotio retinae* (Fig. 265): traumatic oedema
- *Choroidal rupture* (Fig. 266)
- *Retinal tear*: dialysis, equatorial or macular holes may cause retinal detachment
- *Avulsion of the optic nerve*: in severe trauma.

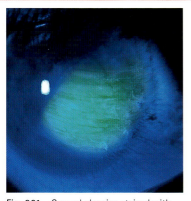

Fig. 261 Corneal abrasion stained with fluorescein.

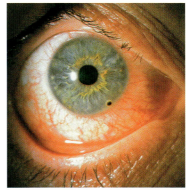

Fig. 262 Corneal foreign body with rust ring.

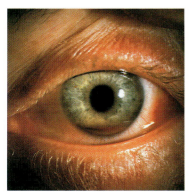

Fig. 263 Hyphaema.

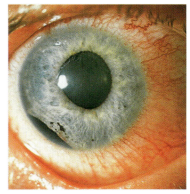

Fig. 264 Iridodialysis.

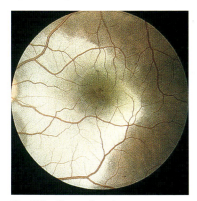

Fig. 265 Commotio retinae.

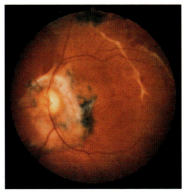

Fig. 266 Choroidal rupture.

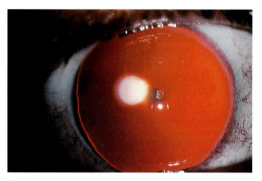

1. This 15-year-old boy was born with the bilateral ocular abnormality shown.

a. What is the diagnosis?
b. Where is the genetic mutation?
c. Some individuals with this condition develop an abdominal tumour. This patient's brother, mother and grandfather all have the eye abnormality shown; what is the likelihood that the patient will develop the tumour?
d. What other ocular features may be present?

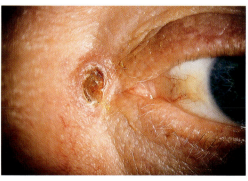

2. This patient is aged 76. The lesion shown has been present for at least a year, its surface intermittently breaks down and crusts.

a. What is the likely diagnosis?
b. What are the different clinical types?
c. What is the treatment?

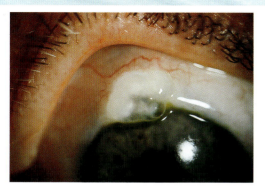

3. This 64-year-old woman recently underwent ocular surgery.

a. What was the surgical procedure?
b. What is the main indication for this operation?
c. What alternative therapy is available?
d. What adjunctive agents can be used if the risk of failure is high?

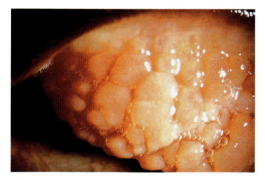

4. This patient has worn rigid contact lenses for 3 years.

a. Describe the signs.
b. What is the histology?
c. What may be the pathogenesis?
d. Give two other causes of this condition.

5. This is a retinal capillary haemangioma.

a. What is the name and inheritance pattern of the phacomatosis associated with this lesion?
b. Name three systemic lesions occurring in this phacomatosis.
c. What proportion of patients with a solitary retinal capillary haemangioma have systemic involvement?
d. How do the retinal lesions threaten sight and how can they be treated?

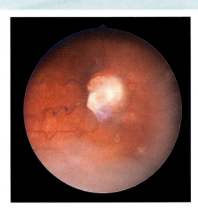

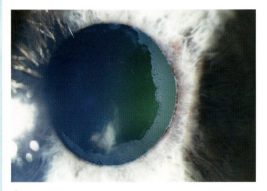

6. A 64-year-old man was found by his optometrist to have this condition in one eye.

a. What is the disorder shown?
b. Approximately what percentage of eyes with this condition develops glaucoma?
c. In which geographical region is it particularly common?
d. Why would cataract surgery be associated with a higher risk of complications?

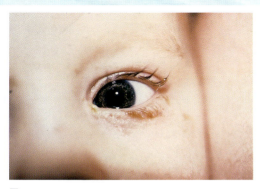

7. The parents of this 6-month-old baby are concerned because the eye has watered persistently since birth.

a. What is the probable cause?
b. What conservative measures might be adopted?
c. At what age should more active intervention be considered, and what form should this take?
d. What is the most important, but much less common, condition that ought to be excluded in an infant with a watering eye?

8. This patient underwent a trabeculectomy 5 days ago.

a. What is the condition shown?
b. What is the likely cause in this context?
c. Clinically, how does the appearance of this condition differ from that of retinal detachment?

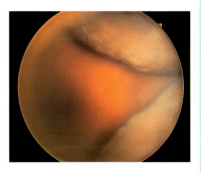

9. This 56-year-old white man first noticed this slowly enlarging brown patch 6 months ago.

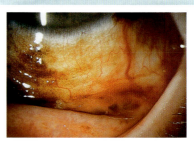

a. What is the diagnosis?
b. What are the two main histological types?
c. Is there any chance of malignant transformation?
d. What are the other causes of diffuse conjunctival pigmentation?

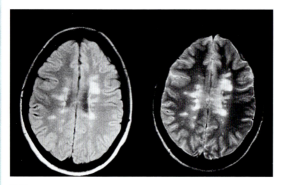

10. This is the MRI scan of a 33-year-old woman who developed blurred vision in the left eye a week ago.

a. What abnormality is shown, and what is the diagnosis?
b. What might be seen on ophthalmoscopy?
c. What other ocular symptoms might she experience during the current episode?
d. What other ocular complications may be associated with this disease?

11. This is a 6-year-old child with orbital cellulitis.

a. What are the life-threatening complications?

b. List alternative diagnostic possibilities.

c. What is the management?

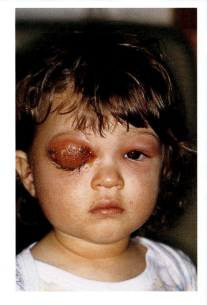

12. This is the fundus of a 36-year-old man who has had type 1 diabetes for 20 years.

a. What grade of diabetic retinopathy is shown?

b. What are the signs of the other grades of diabetic retinopathy?

c. What are the most important risk factors for diabetic retinopathy?

d. List the other ocular complications of diabetes.

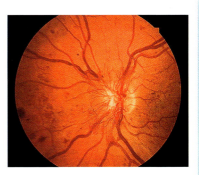

13. This is the fundus of a 72-year-old man with type 2 diabetes.

a. What does the fundus show?
b. Define the three categories of 'clinically significant macular oedema' (CSMO).
c. How is CSMO treated?
d. List factors conferring an adverse prognosis.

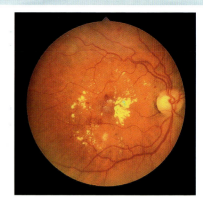

14. This is a choroidal naevus.

a. What clinical features might arouse suspicion that a naevus may be a small melanoma?
b. What treatment modalities are available for melanoma?
c. What factors influence prognosis?

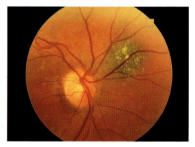

15. This is a 17-year-old boy with epilepsy.

a. What are the facial lesions called?
b. What is the systemic condition in which they are seen, and what is its inheritance pattern?
c. What are the ophthalmic features of the disease?

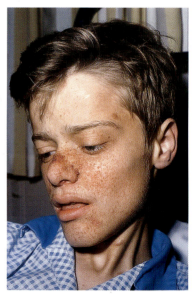

16. This is the fundal appearance of a 70-year-old hypertensive woman.

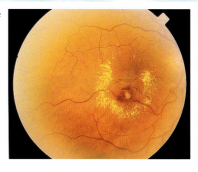

a. What is the lesion?
b. What complications may occur?
c. What is the management?

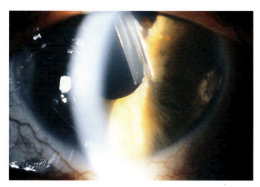

17. This is a glaucoma drainage device.

a. What are the indications for such a device?
b. What proportion of patients undergoing implantation achieves adequate pressure control without additional medication?
c. What are the complications of implantation?

18. This is the bilateral fundal appearance of a 25-year old man. Visual acuity in the right eye is 6/36 and in the left 6/18.

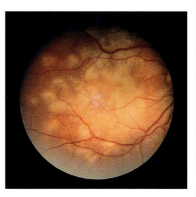

a. Fluorescein angiography shows early hypofluorescence and late hyperfluorescence of the lesions. What is the most likely diagnosis?
b. What other ocular findings may be evident?
c. What systemic features may be present?
d. What is the prognosis?

19. This is the coronal CT scan of a 19-year-old man.

a. What is the abnormality demonstrated?
b. What may be the cause?
c. What physical signs may be present?
d. What is the management?

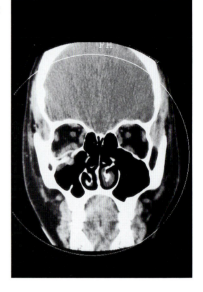

20. This is the fundal appearance in a patient with Grönblad–Strandberg syndrome.

a. What abnormality is shown?
b. What is the histopathology of the lesions?
c. What is *'peau d'orange'* in this context?
d. What are the other systemic associations?

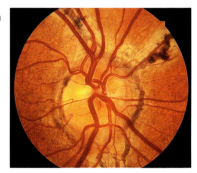

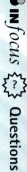

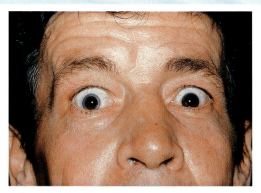

21. This is a 72-year-old patient with Parinaud's (dorsal midbrain) syndrome, showing failure of upgaze.

a. What are the other clinical signs of Parinaud's syndrome?
b. What are the likely causes in a patient of this age?
c. What are the important causes in children?

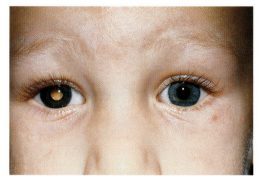

22. The parents of this 18-month-old baby noticed this abnormality.

a. What is this sign called?
b. What is the most important cause to be considered in a child of this age?
c. List the other important causes.

23. This shows herpes zoster ophthalmicus.

a. Describe the evolution of the rash.
b. What is Hutchinson's sign and what is its significance?
c. What are the important ocular complications?

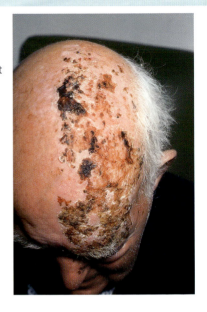

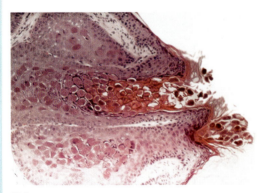

24. This shows the histopathology of a skin lesion caused by a virus.

a. Describe the features and give the diagnosis.
b. What is the characteristic mode of ocular presentation of this condition?
c. Patients with what systemic disease characteristically develop multiple lesions of this type?

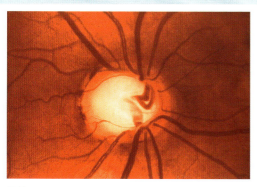

25. This is the optic disc of an 81-year-old man whose intraocular pressure is 12.

a. What is the most likely diagnosis?
b. What systemic features may be present?
c. What are the characteristic visual field defects in this condition?

26. This patient is about to undergo cataract surgery.

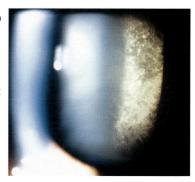

a. What is the morphological type of this lens opacity?
b. Although corrected visual acuity is 6/9, symptoms are substantial. What form are these likely to take?
c. The patient, who is aged only 46, has asthma. What connection might this have with the cataract?

27. This is the fundal appearance of a 37-year-old Turk, who has experienced recurrent mouth ulcers and lower limb arthralgia.

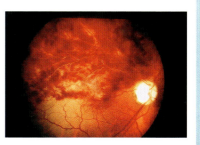

a. What is the ocular diagnosis?
b. What is the probable systemic diagnosis?
c. He has been treated previously for anterior uveitis with hypopyon. Is this significant?
d. What is the likely HLA association?

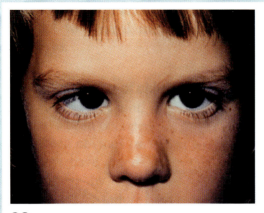

28. A few months ago, the parents of this 4-year-old child noticed that one eye turns in towards the nose.

a. What points should be covered in the history?
b. How should the child be assessed initially?
c. What is the management of convergent squint presenting at this age?

29. This is the fundal appearance of a 63-year-old woman who recently became aware of a small missing patch in the centre of the vision in one eye.

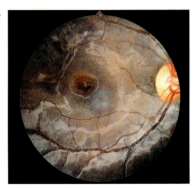

a. What is the diagnosis?
b. What is the visual acuity likely to be?
c. Can anything be done to improve her vision?
d. What is the chance of the condition affecting the other eye?

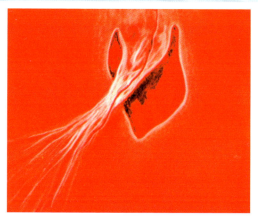

30. This patient experienced the sudden onset of floaters.

a. What abnormality is shown?
b. How should it be treated?
c. What conditions predispose to the development of retinal detachment?

31. This patient has had a photophobic, red and gritty eye for 2 days.

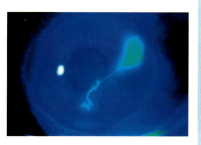

a. What is the diagnosis?
b. What key physical sign should be checked prior to measuring the intraocular pressure?
c. What is the differential diagnosis?
d. What is the treatment?

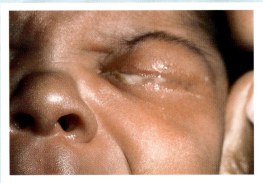

32. The eyes of this 2-week-old baby have been very sticky for the last week.

a. By definition, what is the diagnosis?
b. What are the causes, and when does each typically present?
c. What are the systemic manifestations of chlamydial infection in neonates?

33. This is the fluorescein angiogram of a 70-year-old woman.

a. What lesion is demonstrated?
b. Given the patient's age, what is the likely cause?
c. What other underlying pathology might be responsible?

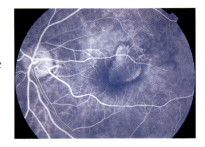

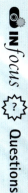

Hess screen chart
Field of left eye (fixing with right eye)

Name.................. No ....
Field of right eye (fixing with left eye)

temp ◄

► Nasal ◄

► temp

Green before left eye

Green before right eye

Diagnosis

34. This is the Hess chart of a 48-year-old patient with double vision.

a. What is the diagnosis?
b. Describe in detail the changes shown on the chart.

35. This is the fundal appearance of a patient who lost vision in the eye earlier in the day.

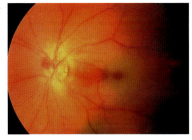

a. Describe the signs.
b. What is the diagnosis?
c. What imaging investigations might be appropriate and why?
d. What are the other common causes of sudden, profound, painless unilateral loss of vision?

36. This patient's optometrist was concerned that this might be a melanoma.

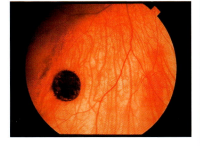

a. What is the diagnosis?
b. What are the characteristics that support this?
c. Are you concerned regarding systemic implications?

37. This patient has had increasing difficulty with night vision (nyctalopia) over the last few years.

a. What are the signs and what is the diagnosis?
b. What other ocular features may be present?
c. What are the electrodiagnostic findings?
d. What systemic disorders may be associated with this condition?

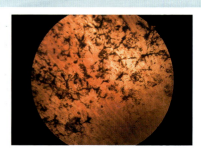

38. This patient has noticed that she sweats much more on one side of her face.

a. Describe the signs and give the diagnosis.
b. What other ocular features may be present?
c. What pharmacological tests might be useful?

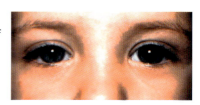

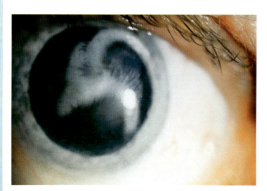

39. This is the cornea of an elderly patient with congenital syphilis.

a. What is the condition?
b. Rarely, an intrastromal corneal haemorrhage may occur. What is the mechanism?
c. List the late systemic signs of congenital syphilis.

40. This patient has long, spindly fingers (arachnodactyly) and a high-arched palate.

a. What is the ocular sign?
b. What is the systemic diagnosis, and what is its genetic basis?
c. What other systemic features may be present?
d. What other systemic conditions are associated with this ocular finding?

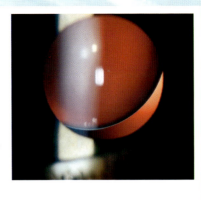

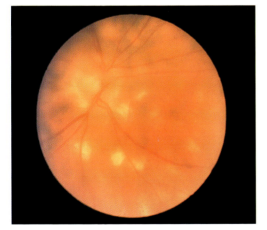

41. This is the retinal appearance in a 56-year-old woman with birdshot retinochoroidopathy.

a. What is the HLA association?
b. Is vitritis common in this condition?
c. What special investigation is useful when deciding to start treatment?
d. What are the most common causes of visual loss?

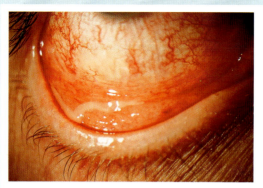

42. This is the eye of a man in his twenties who recently contracted urethritis. Reiter's syndrome is suspected.

a. What other systemic features might he have?
b. What other ocular feature is characteristic?
c. What blood test will help to confirm the diagnosis?
d. What cardiac complication can occur?

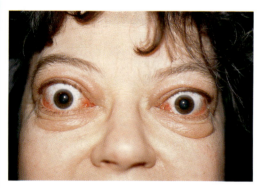

43. This woman aged 40 has thyroid eye disease.

a. What are the symptoms of this condition?
b. Is thyroid eye disease more commonly associated with primary hypo- or hyperthyroidism?
c. What is the least common ocular motility defect?
d. Orbital soft tissue swelling can sometimes lead to optic neuropathy. What treatments are available?

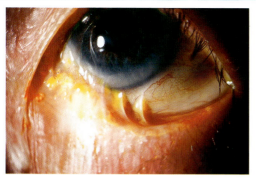

44. This middle-aged woman has ocular cicatricial pemphigoid.

a. What are the typical cutaneous lesions?
b. What are the complications?
c. How is the active disease treated?

45. This is the bilateral optic disc appearance of an obese 30-year-old woman complaining of headache, nausea and transient visual obscurations.

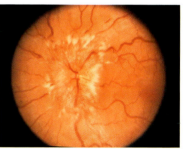

a. What is the likely diagnosis?
b. What is the most important complication?
c. What are the treatment options?

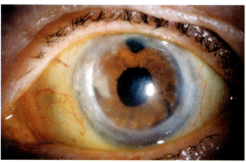

46. This patient underwent penetrating keratoplasty a year ago. For the past month vision in the eye has been blurred as a result of graft failure.

a. Clinically, how does graft failure differ from rejection?
b. How is rejection treated?
c. List factors conferring a poor prognosis for corneal grafting.

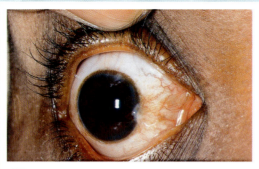

47. This patient has been working in the Middle East for several years.

a. What is the lesion?
b. What are the indications for its removal?
c. What are the possible surgical techniques?

48. At a routine sight test, an optometrist discovered this condition (a fluorescein angiogram is shown) in both eyes of an asymptomatic hypermetropic patient.

a. What is the diagnosis?
b. What is the cause?
c. List other causes.

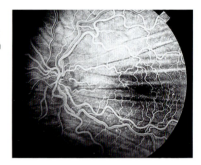

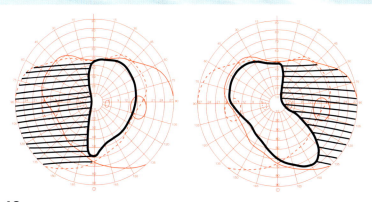

49. These are the visual fields of a 50-year-old woman with a family history of glaucoma but normal intraocular pressures.

a. Are the visual fields typically glaucomatous?
b. What other pathology might be suspected?
c. What other investigation is indicated?

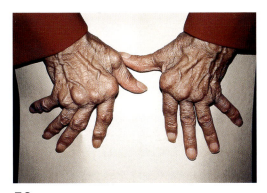

50. This woman has chronic arthritis and complains of persistently gritty eyes.

a. What is the systemic diagnosis?
b. Why are her eyes gritty?
c. What simple tests can help to confirm the diagnosis?
d. What other ocular complications may occur?

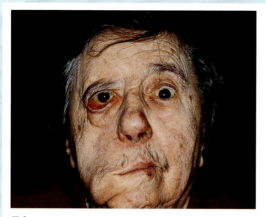

51. This patient underwent removal of an acoustic neuroma 2 weeks ago.

a. What is the abnormality shown?
b. What ocular problems may develop?
c. What is the management?

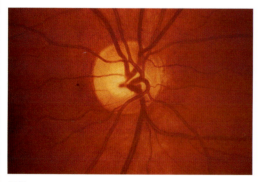

52. This 57-year-old man has intraocular pressures of 26 mmHg in both eyes.

a. Does he have glaucoma?
b. What percentage of patients with this intraocular pressure develop glaucoma?
c. How will measuring the optic disc diameter help to determine if the nerve is normal?
d. What other investigations may be useful?

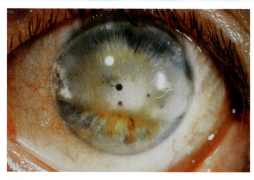

53. This 9-year-old girl suffers from juvenile idiopathic arthritis (JIA).

a. What are the signs shown?
b. What are the ocular manifestations of JIA?
c. List three characteristics in JIA which are associated with a high risk of eye problems.

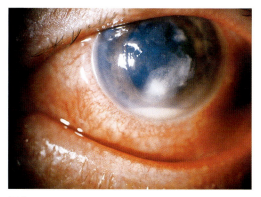

54. This is the cornea of a patient who wears soft contact lenses. The eye has been red and very uncomfortable for 24 hours.

a. What is the diagnosis?
b. What is the management?
c. List the causative microorganisms that do not grow on common culture media but may constitute a serious threat to vision if untreated.

55. (a) The patient is attempting to look to the left; a fine nystagmus can be seen in the left eye. (b) No abnormality is seen on right gaze. (c) Convergence is normal.

a. What is the diagnosis?
b. Where is the lesion located?
c. Give the most likely cause in this patient.
d. List other causes.

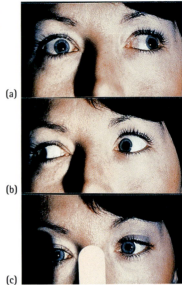

(a)

(b)

(c)

56. This 37-year-old man has granulomatous iritis. Ophthalmoscopy revealed moderate vitritis and retinitis, as shown.

a. He has no risk factors for HIV infection. What is the probable diagnosis?
b. What investigations might help to confirm the diagnosis?
c. What is the management?

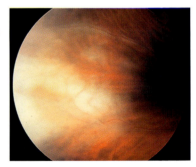

57. This patient sustained an ischaemic central retinal vein occlusion 3 months ago.

a. What complication has occurred, and what is the likely sequel?
b. List other common causes of the condition shown.
c. How should this patient be managed?

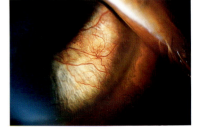

58. This elderly woman presented to the general accident and emergency department with abdominal pain and nausea. The casualty officer noticed that she had a red eye.

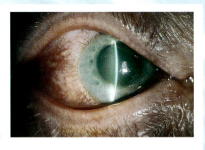

a. What is the diagnosis?
b. What is the management?
c. What are the other common causes of a very painful and red eye?

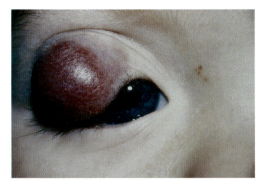

59. This baby's parents are concerned that this rapidly growing lesion may damage the child's eyesight.

a. What is the diagnosis?
b. Is the parents' concern justified?
c. What is the most common form of treatment?
d. Does the lesion have any systemic implications?

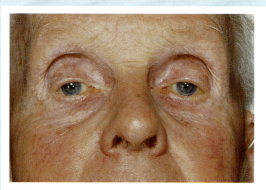

60. Bilateral ptosis is shown.

a. What are the muscles responsible for elevating the upper lid, and what is their innervation?

b. What are the causes of ptosis?

c. What are the causes of pseudoptosis?

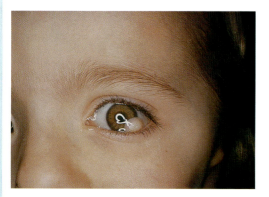

61. This infant's parents are extremely worried by this lesion.

a. What is the diagnosis?

b. What is its pathological categorization?

c. When might treatment be indicated?

d. Are there any systemic implications?

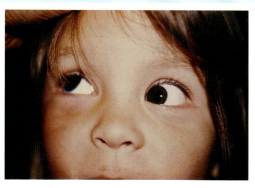

62. This child is attempting to look up and to the right.

a. Describe the motility abnormality and give the diagnosis, assuming eye movements are normal in other positions of gaze.
b. What is the management?
c. Most cases are congenital but what are the causes of an acquired lesion of this type?

63. This elderly patient suddenly lost vision in one eye. Ophthalmoscopy revealed a pale, swollen optic disc.

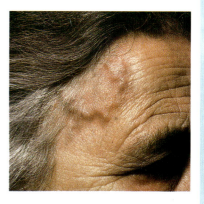

a. What questions are essential in a patient presenting with sudden loss of vision and this disc appearance?
b. What urgent blood tests are indicated?
c. What further investigation is necessary?

64. This child also has ptosis and progressive bilateral extraocular muscle weakness.

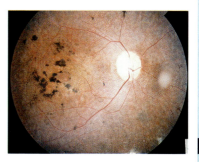

a. What is the diagnosis?
b. What is the underlying genetic abnormality?
c. In addition to genetic analysis, what investigations might be helpful in confirmation of the diagnosis?

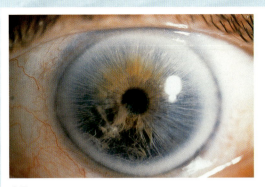

65. This 78-year-old man has bilateral corneal arcus as well as this condition in both eyes.

a. What is the diagnosis?
b. How is sight threatened?
c. What is the treatment?

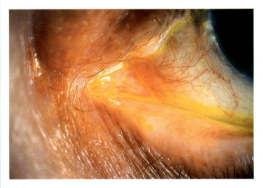

66. This 60-year-old woman complains of watering of the eye for the last 6 months.

a. What abnormality is shown?
b. What further investigations should be performed to exclude other causes of the watering?
c. Assuming the abnormality above is responsible for the symptoms, what are the treatment options?

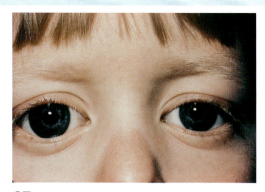

67. This child was born with the condition shown.

a. Describe the signs; what is the likely diagnosis?
b. What other signs might be present in this condition?
c. How can the diagnosis be confirmed?

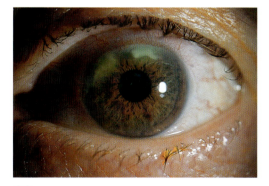

68. This 33–year–old man complains of mild ocular irritation for the last 3 days.

a. What is the diagnosis?
b. What features suggest that this is not a bacterial keratitis?
c. What is the treatment?

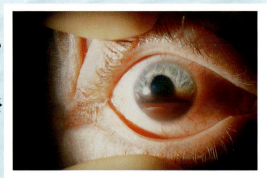

69. This 15-year-old boy was struck in the eye by a tennis ball.

a. What is the sign shown?
b. What is the most important complication of this condition?
c. What management should be instituted?

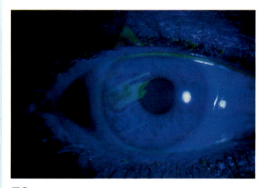

70. This patient was poked in the eye by a baby earlier in the day.

a. What is this lesion?
b. What are the symptoms?
c. What is the management?

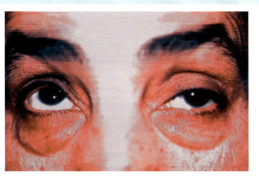

71. This 50-year-old suddenly developed a droopy eyelid and double vision associated with ipsilateral frontal headache.

a. What is the diagnosis?
b. What underlying condition must be urgently excluded?
c. What clinical features are important when considering the cause?

72. This patient recently underwent retinal detachment surgery.

a. The complication of retinal detachment shown is the most common cause of failure of surgical repair. What is it?
b. List the signs of the condition.
c. What form of surgery is likely to be used to attempt re-attachment?

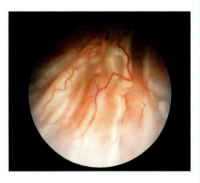

73. This healthy 35-year-old woman presented with the sudden onset of floaters.

a. What is shown?
b. As there is no useful view of the fundus, what investigation should be performed?
c. List the causes of the condition shown.

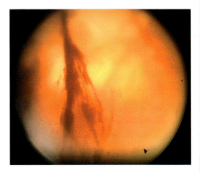

74. This middle-aged patient complains of gradually worsening distortion of vision.

a. What abnormality is shown?
b. What is its histopathological basis?
c. What are the causes?

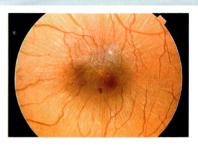

75. These are instrumentation used to perform pars plana vitrectomy (PPV).

a. Name the instruments.
b. List the important indications for PPV.

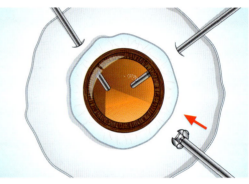

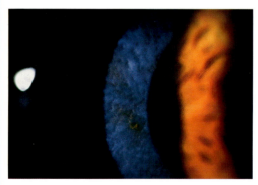

76. This patient has grey-white round and polygonal opacities in the superficial cornea, densest centrally and forming a honeycomb pattern in places; the diagnosis is Thiel–Behnke corneal dystrophy (Bowman layer dystrophy type 2).

a. What is the typical clinical presentation of this condition?
b. Describe the histology.
c. What is the inheritance pattern and where is the gene?
d. What is the other dystrophy affecting the Bowman layer and how do the two differ clinically?

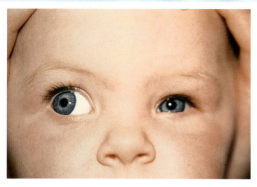

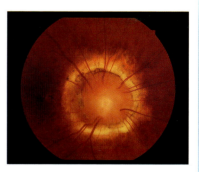

77. This boy with a congenital ocular motility disorder is attempting right gaze.

a. Describe the signs and give the diagnosis.
b. How would he be categorized in the Huber classification of this disorder?
c. Excluding other motility signs, what are the ocular associations of this condition?

78. Vision is very poor in this eye; the fellow eye is normal.

a. Describe the signs and give the diagnosis.
b. What is the incidence of subsequent serous retinal detachment?
c. What are the systemic implications?

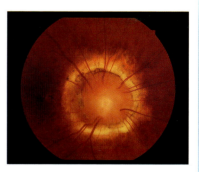

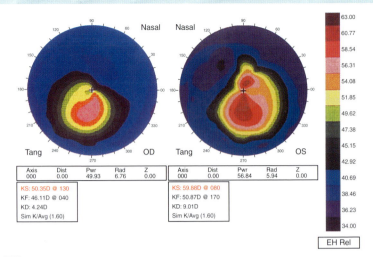

79. This investigation was used to assess the cornea of a 23-year-old woman with increasing astigmatism.

a. What was the investigation employed?
b. What is represented by the colour coding used?
c. Is the cornea normal according to the scan?

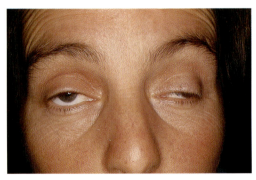

80. This patient complains of drooping eyelids worse towards the end of the day together with intermittent double vision.

a. What underlying systemic disease may be present?
b. What other eye signs would reinforce the putative diagnosis?
c. What blood test can be useful in helping to confirm the diagnosis?
d. What pharmacological test might be indicated?

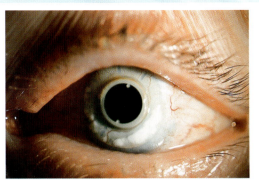

81. This patient sustained a severe bilateral chemical injury 3 years ago.

a. What is the device shown?
b. What are the indications for surgery of this type?
c. What are the complications?

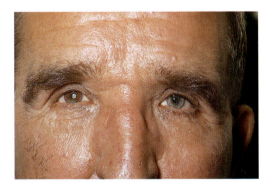

82. This man has noticed worsening vision in the right eye over the past few months. Diffuse stellate keratic precipitates are present on slit lamp examination.

a. Describe the signs and give the diagnosis.
b. Besides that shown, what other sight-threatening complications might occur?
c. How is the condition treated?

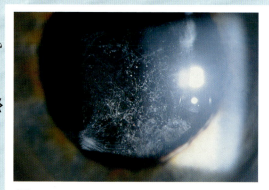

83. The vision in this pseudophakic eye has gradually been getting worse for several months.

a. Describe the complication of cataract surgery shown.
b. What other symptoms is the patient likely to be experiencing?
c. What is the treatment?
d. What are the complications of the treatment?

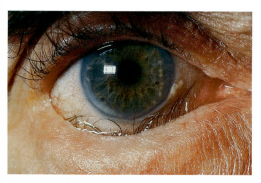

84. This patient's eye has been gritty and red for several weeks.

a. What is the cause of the symptoms?
b. What is the pathogenesis of the involutional form of this condition?
c. What is the treatment?

85. This 81-year-old woman has severe 'wet' age-related macular degeneration in her other eye. Her optometrist was concerned about a recent fall in the vision of the eye shown above.

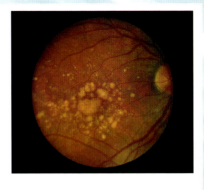

a. What is the condition shown?
b. If there is clinical suspicion of choroidal neovascularization (CNV), what investigation should be performed?
c. Is there anything that can be done to reduce the risk of CNV in this eye?

86. This elderly patient has a dome-shaped macular elevation corresponding to the abnormality shown above.

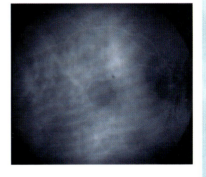

a. What is the investigation shown?
b. What is the lesion?
c. What is the pathogenesis?
d. How might it be treated?

87. This 16-year-old girl has been unwell for several weeks. A physician identified this fundal appearance.

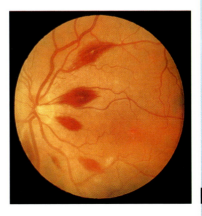

a. Describe the lesions. What are they called?
b. Leukaemia is a possible underlying diagnosis. List others.
c. How else might leukaemia manifest in the eyes?

88. This patient has oculocutaneous albinism with white hair and very pale skin.

a. Is he likely to be tyrosinase-negative or -positive?
b. How would visual-evoked potential analysis help in the assessment of this patient?
c. Name two systemic syndromes associated with this condition.
d. Could this patient have either of these syndromes?

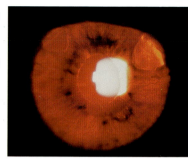

89. This was an incidental finding in a 30-year-old man.

a. Describe the lesion. What is the most likely cause?
b. At what age do such lesions tend to reactivate in immunocompetent individuals?
c. What diagnostic tests are available?

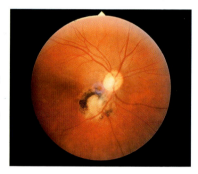

90. This patient recently underwent cataract surgery complicated by vitreous loss.

a. What is shown?
b. What is meant by 'vitreous loss'?
c. What are the postoperative complications of vitreous loss?

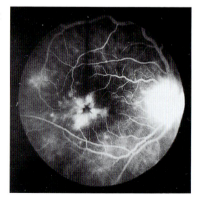

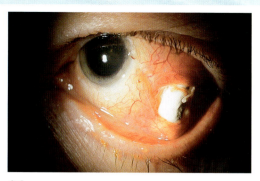

91. Retinal detachment surgery involving placement of an explant was carried out on this patient's eye 1 year ago.

a. What complication has occurred?
b. Could removal of the explant precipitate re-detachment?
c. How should the explant be removed?

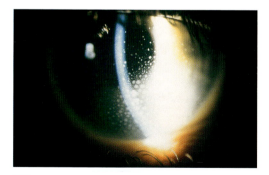

92. This patient presented with a sore red eye.

a. What sign is present?
b. The patient has had no previous eye problems and is otherwise healthy. Is systemic investigation indicated?
c. What screening investigations might be carried out?

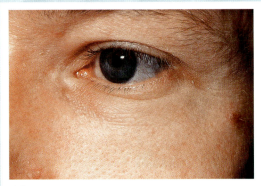

93. This patient has a systemic disorder associated with multiple fractures and deafness.

a. What is the systemic disorder?
b. What is the pathological basis of the abnormality shown?
c. What other systemic diseases are associated with this sign?

94. This patient has approximately 10 dioptres of myopia.

a. What is the pathological process shown?
b. List other ocular associations of high myopia.
c. Is this patient's ocular axial length likely to be nearer 20 mm or 30 mm?

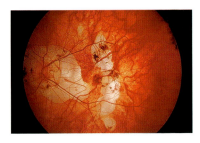

95. This myopic patient is undergoing refractive surgery.

a. What is the procedure?
b. Can this procedure also be used to correct hypermetropia or astigmatism?
c. What complications may occur?

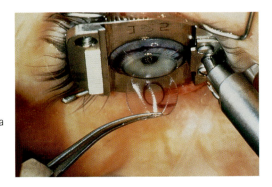

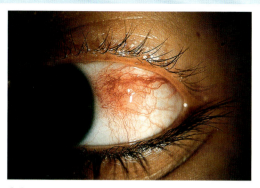

96. This 30-year-old woman has been aware of this triangular red patch and mild aching in the eye for 3 days.

a. What is the diagnosis?
b. Classify this condition.
c. Should systemic investigations be performed?
d. What is the treatment?

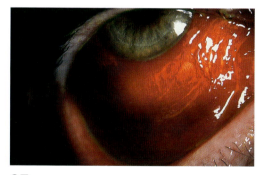

97. While shaving, this patient noticed the appearance shown.

a. What is the diagnosis?
b. What symptoms may be present?
c. What investigations are required?

98. The visual acuity in this 30-year-old man's right eye has deteriorated over the last couple of days.

a. What is the likely diagnosis?
b. What is the visual acuity likely to be?
c. If there is any doubt regarding the diagnosis, what investigation is appropriate?

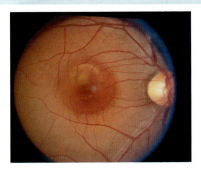

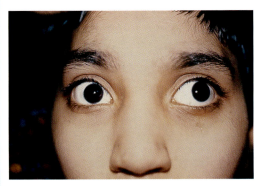

99. This child's left eye turns outward when he is tired, day-dreaming or exposed to bright light.

a. What is the diagnosis?
b. What are the clinical categories of this form of strabismus?
c. How is it managed?

100. This child is undergoing occlusion therapy for amblyopia.

a. What is amblyopia?
b. What are the causes?
c. What is the usual age limit for useful treatment of amblyopia?

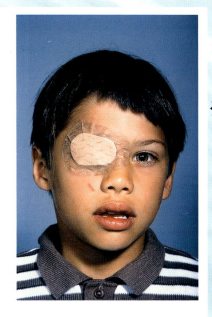

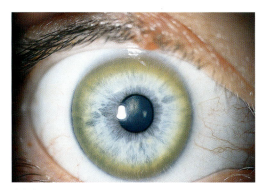

101. This young woman has been undergoing psychiatric investigation; one of her doctors noticed this ocular sign.

a. What is the sign called?
b. What is the histology?
c. What is the underlying diagnosis?
d. What is the other common ocular sign?
e. What are the other major systemic abnormalities?

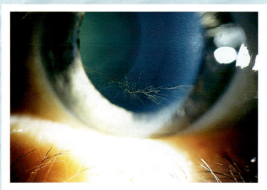

102. This elderly patient takes a drug for cardiac arrhythmia.

a. Describe and name the corneal appearance.
b. What drug is the patient likely to be taking?
c. What proportion of patients on the cardiac drug develop this?
d. What other drugs, and what disease, can give a similar appearance?

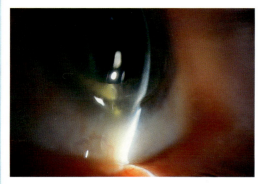

103. This otherwise healthy 55-year-old man has developed increasing astigmatism over several months in both eyes. After an Internet search he wonders whether he has keratoconus.

a. Regardless of the corneal appearance, do you think the patient's diagnosis is correct?
b. What is the significance of the precise location of the changes shown?
c. What is the likely diagnosis?

104. This 40-year-old woman complains that her left eye is gradually getting larger. CT of the orbit showed a well-circumscribed oval lesion within the muscle cone.

a. Bearing in mind the CT finding, what is the sign shown?
b. This lesion is the most common benign orbital tumour in adults; what is the diagnosis?
c. What other ocular signs might be present?
d. What is the treatment?

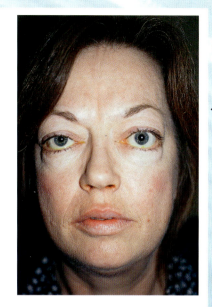

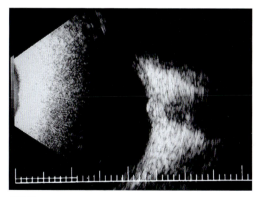

105. Ophthalmological review has been requested by a physician, who is uncertain if this young adult's optic discs are swollen.

a. What is the investigation shown?
b. What abnormality is demonstrated?
c. What other investigations could be performed?

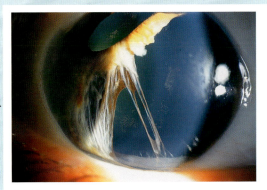

106. This eye of a 35-year-old woman has glaucoma. The fellow eye is normal.

a. What is the likely diagnosis?
b. What are the other forms of this condition?
c. What proportion of patients develop glaucoma?

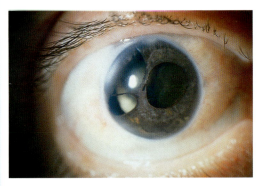

107. This patient has congenital dental and facial anomalies as well as this condition, which affects both eyes.

a. Describe the signs.
b. What is the diagnosis?
c. What is the genetic basis of this condition?
d. What proportion of patients develop glaucoma, and at what age?

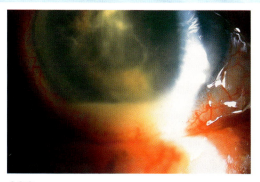

108. Cataract surgery was carried out on this eye 2 days earlier.

a. Describe the signs.
b. What is the probable diagnosis?
c. What is the management?

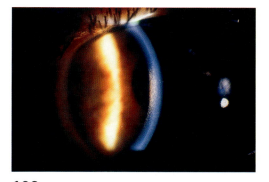

109. A 29-year-old man was found to have this appearance at a routine refraction.

a. What is the sign called?
b. What is the likely diagnosis?
c. What is the probable refractive error?
d. What proportion of patients with this condition are likely to develop glaucoma?

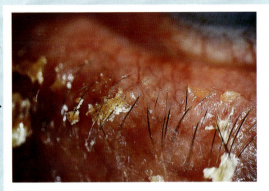

110. Persistent irritation, redness and stickiness, worse in the morning, have led this patient's general practitioner to refer him to an ophthalmologist.

a. What signs are evident?
b. What is the diagnosis?
c. What is the treatment?

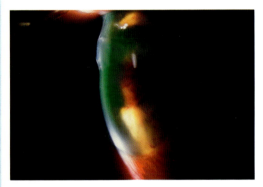

111. This young man was involved in a car accident; he was not wearing a seatbelt.

a. What injury is shown?
b. How should this be managed?

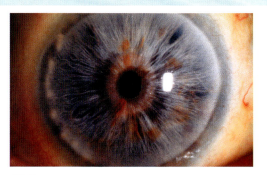

112. This patient with glaucoma described episodic blurring of vision associated with rainbows around lights; the episodes ceased following a laser procedure.

a. What form of laser treatment has been carried out?
b. What forms of glaucoma can present with these symptoms?
c. What other uses are there for the type of laser used to treated this patient?

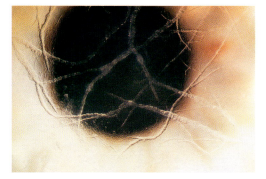

113. This is a symmetrically bilateral appearance in a 51-year-old patient with slowly deteriorating vision.

a. What is the diagnosis?
b. Are recurrent erosions common in this disorder?
c. Will the patient require penetrating keratoplasty?
d. What are the other forms of this disorder?

114. This is the fundus of an 8-week-old baby.

a. What is the diagnosis?
b. Describe the different stages of this disease.
c. What are the criteria for the decision to treat this condition?
d. What form will treatment take?

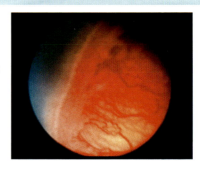

115. This is the fundus appearance in both eyes of a 40-year-old man with severe headaches.

a. What clinical test is indicated?
b. Why are the macular exudates distributed in the fashion shown?
c. What other fundus signs might be seen in this condition?

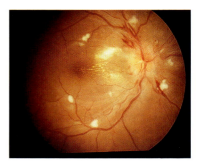

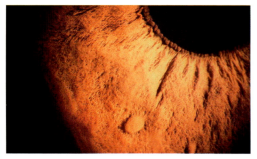

116. This is the iris appearance in a 34-year-old man.

a. What is the sign?
b. What is the probable underlying systemic disease?
c. What are the other ophthalmic features of the systemic disorder?
d. What is the inheritance pattern, and where is the gene locus?

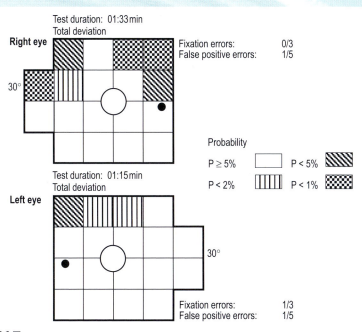

Test duration: 01:33 min
Total deviation

Right eye

30°

Fixation errors: 0/3
False positive errors: 1/5

Probability

P ≥ 5% [ ] P < 5% [hatched]

P < 2% [vertical lines] P < 1% [checkered]

Test duration: 01:15 min
Total deviation

Left eye

30°

Fixation errors: 1/3
False positive errors: 1/5

117. This patient has been referred to the eye clinic by her optician.

a. What is the investigation shown?
b. What is the principle behind the test?
c. What are its main advantages?

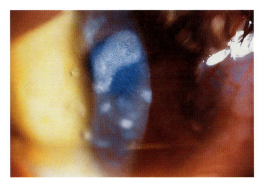

118. This elderly Indian patient has had these whitish corneal nodules for many years.

a. What are the lesions?
b. What is likely to be the underlying eye disease responsible?
c. What is the treatment?

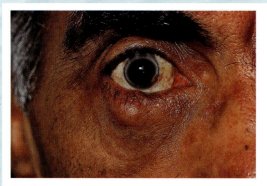

119. This painless lump has been present for several months.

a. What is the diagnosis and pathogenesis?
b. What is the corresponding conjunctival lesion?
c. What forms of treatment are available?

120. The patient's general practitioner was concerned about this fundal appearance.

a. What is the diagnosis?
b. What are the ocular associations?
c. What is the pathogenesis?
d. What is the population prevalence?

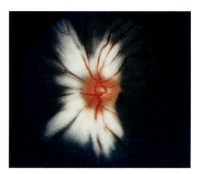

Answers

1.
    a. Aniridia.
    b. Usually in the *PAX6* gene on chromosome 11p13.
    c. Probably the same as the general population. Aniridia is classified into AN-1 (65% of patients) with autosomal dominant inheritance and no systemic implications, AN-2 (33%), a sporadic form carrying a 30% risk of Wilms' tumour (Miller's syndrome), and AN-3 or Gillespie's syndrome with autosomal recessive inheritance, associated with neurological problems.
    d. Nystagmus, glaucoma, cataract, lens subluxation, foveal and optic nerve hypoplasia and corneal opacity.

2.
    a. Basal cell carcinoma (BCC).
    b. Nodulo-ulcerative ('rodent ulcer') and sclerosing types.
    c. Surgical excision, including a wide (4 mm) margin of clinically normal tissue.

3.
    a. Trabeculectomy, a form of filtering surgery.
    b. Glaucoma.
    c. • Topical prostaglandin derivatives, beta-blockers, alpha agonists, carbonic anhydrase inhibitors and miotics.
      • Systemic carbonic anhydrase inhibitors.
      • Laser trabeculoplasty, cyclodiode and peripheral iridotomy in narrow-angle glaucoma.
      • Non-penetrating drainage surgery (e.g. viscocanalostomy) and valve implants (e.g. Molteno).
    d. 5-fluorouracil and mitomycin C.

4.
    a. There are multiple large, highly vascular, cobblestone-like conjunctival projections.
    b. Hyperplastic conjunctival epithelium surrounds a vascular core and a cellular chronic inflammatory infiltrate (lymphocytes, plasma cells, eosinophils).
    c. • Mechanical irritation by a poorly fitting lens.
      • Allergy to lens material or cleaning solutions.
      • Immune reaction to lens deposits.
    d. Severe chronic allergic conjunctivitis and a protruding suture.

5.
    a. Von Hippel–Lindau syndrome (VHL).
    b. CNS haemangioblastoma, renal carcinoma, phaeochromocytoma, polycythaemia, and renal, pancreatic and other abdominal cysts.
    c. Approximately 50%. Virtually all patients with multiple retinal tumours will have VHL.

    d. Most commonly by retinal exudation and occasionally by vitreous haemorrhage and epiretinal membrane formation. The lesions can be treated with laser photocoagulation, cryotherapy or plaque radiotherapy (brachytherapy).

6.
    a. Pseudoexfoliation.
    b. The cumulative risk of developing glaucoma in eyes with pseudoexfoliation is about 5% at 5 years and 15% at 10 years, although this is much higher if the fellow eye already has pseudoexfoliative glaucoma.
    c. Scandinavia.
    d. The pupil frequently dilates poorly, making access to the lens difficult. The lens capsule and zonules are fragile, leading to an increased risk of capsular rupture and vitreous loss. Postoperatively, corneal decompensation and capsular opacification are more common, as is late dislocation of the implant.

7.
    a. Failure of canalization of the nasolacrimal duct.
    b. Daily lacrimal sac massage.
    c. Probing of the lacrimal system should be considered only at 12 months; dacryocystorhinostomy may be necessary in resistant cases.
    d. Congenital glaucoma.

8.
    a. Choroidal detachment.
    b. Overfiltration with associated low intraocular pressure.
    c. A choroidal detachment appears as a smooth, brown convex elevation that does not involve the posterior pole, being limited by the exit points of the vortex veins. The ora serrata does not limit anterior fluid spread, and thus may be visible without indentation.

9.
    a. Primary acquired melanosis (PAM).
    b. PAM with and without atypia, the latter a proliferation of normal melanocytes within the basal epithelial layer, the former shows large melanocytes with prominent nucleoli and pagetoid spread.
    c. About 50% within 5 years in PAM with atypia.
    d. Racial epithelial melanosis and congenital melanocytosis (in contrast to PAM, lies deep to the conjunctiva and cannot be moved over the sclera).

10.
    a. Periventricular demyelinated plaques, their long axes aligned with the ventricular margins; the patient has optic neuritis associated with multiple sclerosis.
    b. The optic disc may be normal (retrobulbar neuritis) or, less commonly, swollen and hyperaemic (papillitis). There may be pallor of the contralateral optic disc, usually temporally. Retinal vascular sheathing is sometimes present.
    c. Pain, particularly on upgaze, headache, tenderness of the eye, decreased colour vision and visual field loss.

d. Ocular motor cranial nerve palsies, internuclear ophthalmoplegia, nystagmus; rarely, intermediate uveitis and peripheral retinal vasculitis.

11.
a. Meningitis, brain abscess and cavernous sinus thrombosis.
b. Preseptal cellulitis, rhabdomyosarcoma and orbital inflammation associated with retinoblastoma and leukaemia.
c. Conjunctival and nasal swabs, intravenous antibiotics and monitoring of optic nerve function. Urgent orbital CT scan to exclude periosteal abscess should be considered. Involve otorhinolaryngological colleagues because sinus washout may be required.

12.
a. Proliferative diabetic retinopathy (DR) with disc neovascularization.
b. Background DR – exudates and dot and blot haemorrhages; preproliferative DR – deep round haemorrhages, cotton wool spots and venous irregularity; advanced DR – vitreous haemorrhage and tractional retinal detachment.
c. Duration of diabetes, poor control, hypertension, renal impairment and obesity. Hyperlipidaemia and smoking may also be important. Pregnancy is sometimes associated with rapid deterioration.
d. Cataract, unstable refraction, ocular motor nerve palsies, neovascular glaucoma, asteroid hyalosis, papillopathy, iris transillumination defects and orbital mucormycosis.

13.
a. Severe background diabetic retinopathy.
b. • Retinal thickening within 500 μm of the centre of the macula.
   • Exudates within 500 μm of the centre of the macula if associated with retinal thickening.
   • Retinal thickening within one disc diameter of the centre of the macula if greater than one disc area in size.
c. With focal argon laser photocoagulation to points of leakage (usually microaneurysms) or grid laser to diffusely leaking areas. Innovative modalities include intravitreal steroids, systemic pharmaceutical agents and vitrectomy.
d. Hard exudates involving the fovea, significant ischaemia, diffuse rather than focal oedema, cystoid macular oedema and poor visual acuity at presentation.

14.
a. Visual symptoms, especially photopsia. Large lesion size: diameter >5 mm, thickness >1 mm, orange pigment overlying the lesion, associated subretinal fluid and documented increase in size after puberty.
b. Largely dependent on patient profile (especially age), tumour size and location and preferences of the patient and surgeon. Modalities available for the primary tumour include radioactive plaque application (brachytherapy), external beam radiotherapy, local resection, enucleation, stereotactic radiosurgery using the gamma knife and diode laser transpupillary thermotherapy ('TTT').

c. Histological type, the presence of chromosomal abnormalities in tumour cells, tumour size, patient age, the presence or absence of extrascleral extension and tumour location (anterior worse than posterior).

15.   a. Adenoma sebaceum.

b. Tuberous sclerosis, also known as Bourneville's disease, which is inherited in an autosomal dominant pattern.

c. Retinal astrocytomas are present in about 50%. Other rarer features include the ocular sequelae of raised intracranial pressure (papilloedema, optic atrophy and sixth nerve paresis) and hypopigmented retinal and iris spots.

16.   a. A retinal artery macroaneurysm.

b. Frequently, these lesions thrombose and undergo spontaneous involution. However, chronic leakage may cause retinal oedema, with the risk of macular involvement. Haemorrhage may occur if the macroaneurysm ruptures.

c. Laser may be applied to a vision-threatening lesion, otherwise observation is appropriate.

17.   a. Artificial drainage shunts are used when the success rate of trabeculectomy is low. Examples include neovascular, traumatic and certain developmental glaucomas, severe conjunctival scarring and uncontrolled glaucoma despite previous trabeculectomy with adjunctive antimetabolite.

b. Only about one-third in the longer term.

c. Overdrainage (with shallow/flat anterior chamber), cataract, corneal decompensation, tube retraction or erosion through the conjunctiva, endophthalmitis and extraocular muscle imbalance.

18.   a. Acute multifocal posterior placoid pigment epitheliopathy (AMPPPE).

b. Iritis and vitritis, and sometimes optic disc oedema and retinal periphlebitis.

c. An influenza-like illness and erythema nodosum.

d. The prognosis is good, 80% of eyes regaining 6/12 or better.

19.   a. The scan shows a right orbital floor 'blowout' fracture.

b. Severe blunt trauma.

c. Periocular swelling and bruising, subcutaneous air ('surgical emphysema'), enophthalmos, paraesthesia in the infraorbital nerve distribution, limitation of vertical eye movement and damage to the globe.

d. Systemic antibiotics (as this is a compound fracture), avoidance of blowing the nose, and surgical repair if indicated, usually for larger defects and soft tissue entrapment; timing of surgery is controversial.

20.   a. Angioid streaks; the combination of these and pseudoxanthoma elasticum is known as Grönblad–Strandberg syndrome.

b. Angioid streaks consist of dehiscences in the elastic layer of the Bruch membrane due to progressive degeneration and deposition of calcium with secondary changes in the retinal pigment epithelium and choriocapillaris.

c. *Peau d'orange* ('orange skin'), refers to a pigmented mottling, particularly evident temporal to the macula, seen in eyes with angioid streaks.

d. Ehlers–Danlos syndrome type 6, Paget's disease and possibly certain haemoglobinopathies.

21.
a. Light–near dissociation of pupillary reactions, lid retraction (Collier's sign), convergence–retraction nystagmus (elicited with an optokinetic nystagmus drum), paresis (or spasm) of convergence and accommodation. Downgaze is typically normal. The eyes will be straight in the primary position of gaze in the absence of additional motility abnormality.

b. Stroke or tumour involving the midbrain and posterior fossa aneurysm.

c. Sylvian aqueduct stenosis, pinealoma and meningitis.

22.
a. Leukocoria: 'white pupil'.

b. Retinoblastoma, the most common malignant intraocular tumour in children; 60% of cases present with leukoria and both eyes are affected in 30% of patients.

c. Persistent hyperplastic primary vitreous, Coats' disease, advanced retinopathy of prematurity and toxocariasis.

23.
a. An initial maculopapular rash progresses to form vesicles and subsequently crusting ulcers; associated periorbital oedema is typical.

b. This refers to skin lesions on the side of the tip of the nose and is associated with an increased risk of ocular complications.

c. Acute iritis, keratitis (epithelial, nummular, disciform and neurotrophic), scleritis, optic neuritis and ocular motor nerve palsies.

24.
a. A well-defined nodule with a central crater. The base consists of proliferating squamous cells with eosinophilic cytoplasmic inclusions that enlarge as they progress towards the large central crater, degenerating with loss of their nuclei in the process. The diagnosis is molluscum contagiosum.

b. With a persistent follicular conjunctivitis, caused by continual shedding of viral particles from a lesion on the lid margin.

c. Acquired immune deficiency syndrome (AIDS).

25.
a. Normal-tension glaucoma because the disc shows glaucomatous cupping.

b. A range of vascular phenomena have been reported: Raynaud's phenomenon, migraine, nocturnal systemic hypotension, reduced blood flow velocity of the ophthalmic and ciliary arteries, paraproteinaemia and the presence of serum autoantibodies.

c. Paracentral scotoma, nasal step, arcuate defect, ring scotoma and end-stage with a small residual central island.

26. a. Posterior subcapsular (PSC).
   b. Symptoms out of proportion to the corrected visual acuity such as substantial glare, vision worse in bright light or when encountering car headlights at night, and difficulty with reading vision, caused by pupillary constriction enhancing the effect of the opacity.
   c. The patient may have taken systemic steroids, which promote the formation of PSC cataract.

27. a. Superotemporal branch retinal vein occlusion.
   b. Behçet's disease. A retinal venous occlusion is very uncommon in a patient of this age without an underlying predisposing condition. Behçet's affects the venous circulation more than the arterial.
   c. Yes; anterior uveitis, often with a hypopyon, is one of the major diagnostic criteria for Behçet's, along with recurrent aphthous oral ulceration.
   d. HLA-B51.

28. a. Besides age of onset and variability of the squint, family history, birth history and general health.
   b. Visual acuity, stereopsis, confirm the presence of a deviation (i.e. exclude pseudoesotropia), measurement of the deviation, checking the ocular movements (particularly to exclude a sixth nerve palsy), refraction and ocular examination (a squint can be the presenting sign of pathology such as retinoblastoma and congenital cataract).
   c. Typically, a hypermetropic refractive error will be present. Spectacle correction will usually partially or completely control the squint, and the child should be reviewed after several weeks.

29. a. Age-related macular hole.
   b. Typically this will be 6/60, though eccentric fixation may permit up to 6/9.
   c. Vitrectomy, usually accompanied by peeling of the internal limiting membrane surrounding the hole, and intraocular gas injection, facilitates closure of the hole and visual improvement in most patients. Best results are achieved with holes present for less than a year.
   d. Up to 15% at 5 years.

30. a. A U-shaped retinal tear.
   b. Laser photocoagulation with two rows of confluent burns. If the tear is very peripheral, cryotherapy may be easier to apply.
   c. Myopia, lattice degeneration, aphakia and pseudophakia (particularly when complicated by vitreous loss), trauma (old or recent), and family history of retinal detachment, especially when associated with Stickler's syndrome.

31.

   a. Dendritic ulcer due to herpes simplex keratitis (HSK).

   b. Corneal sensation is typically reduced in HSK and must be checked before the instillation of local anaesthetic.

   c. Healing corneal abrasion is probably the most common source of diagnostic difficulty; other causes of a dendritic appearance include herpes zoster keratitis, the epitheliopathy of contact lens wear, acanthamoeba keratitis and topical medication toxicity.

   d. Topical aciclovir, ganciclovir or trifluorothymidine. Debridement is used in some circumstances. Long-term oral aciclovir can be used to reduce the frequency of recurrence if necessary.

32.

   a. Neonatal conjunctivitis or 'ophthalmia neonatorum' – conjunctivitis occurring within the first neonatal month.

   b. • Chemical conjunctivitis: within the first postnatal week is usually due to antiseptic agents although in the past commonly due to silver nitrate gonococcus prophylaxis.

      • Gonococcus: within the first week.

      • Chlamydia: 1–3 weeks

      • Herpes simplex: 1–2 weeks

      • Staphylococci and other bacteria: end of first week onwards.

   c. Infection may involve the lungs (pneumonitis), nasopharynx, middle ear, vagina and rectum.

33.

   a. Although a series of frames is ideally required to ascertain the diagnosis, this almost certainly shows a choroidal neovascular membrane.

   b. The 'wet' form of age-related macular degeneration.

   c. Other, less common, causes include myopia, punctate inner choroidopathy, traumatic choroidal rupture, angioid streaks, inappropriate retinal laser photocoagulation and optic disc drusen.

34.

   a. Right superior oblique palsy.

   b. The smaller area is enclosed by the chart for the right eye, suggesting that this is the abnormal side. The right chart is centred at a higher level than the left, showing that this is the higher eye in the primary position. In addition to the primary underaction of the right superior oblique, there is overaction (due to contracture with time) of the unopposed ipsilateral inferior oblique, overaction of the contralateral inferior rectus yoke muscle (due to Hering's law of equal innervation), and underaction of the contralateral superior rectus (due to Hering's law, as the contracted right inferior oblique requires less innervation).

35.

   a. The retina appears pale and oedematous, except at the centre of the macula where the contrast gives the appearance of a 'cherry-red spot'. The arterioles are attenuated.

   b. Central retinal artery occlusion.

   c. Carotid artery assessment by ultrasound (duplex), MRI or conventional angiography, and cardiac imaging, in order to exclude an embolic source.

d. Vitreous haemorrhage, branch retinal artery occlusion, retinal venous occlusion, macular haemorrhage (usually due to macular degeneration), anterior ischaemic optic neuropathy and optic neuritis.

36.
a. The 'typical' form of congenital hypertrophy of the retinal pigment epithelium (CHRPE).
b. The lesion is solitary, flat, dark-grey to black, round, with a hypopigmented rim and hypopigmented lacunae.
c. The 'typical' form of CHRPE does not carry any systemic implications, in contrast to the 'atypical' form (spindle-shaped or oval, multiple, bilateral, hypopigmentation at one margin), which is associated with familial adenomatous polyposis, Gardner's syndrome and Turcot's syndrome.

37.
a. Mid-peripheral retinal pigmentary deposits in a bone-spicule pattern, waxy disc pallor and arteriolar attenuation, characteristic of retinitis pigmentosa.
b. Relatively common features include: mid-periphery annular scotomas, maculopathy (cystoid oedema, atrophy), posterior subcapsular cataracts, myopia and open-angle glaucoma (3%).
c. Reduced scotopic (and later photopic) responses in ERG, abnormal EOG, prolonged dark adaptation.
d. Important conditions include Bassen–Kornzweig syndrome, Refsum's syndrome, Usher's syndrome, Kearns–Sayre syndrome and Bardet–Biedl syndrome.

38.
a. Slight right ptosis and miosis. The diagnosis is Horner's syndrome. The patient is actually experiencing reduced sweating on the abnormal side, as the lesion is proximal to the splitting of the sudomotor fibres to travel along the external carotid.
b. Slight elevation of the lower eyelid, heterochromia, relative hypotony, conjunctival hyperaemia and hyperaccommodation.
c. Cocaine 4% dilates a normal pupil due to prevention of noradrenaline (norepinephrine) re-uptake, but not a Horner's pupil. Hydroxyamphetamine 1% causes release of noradrenaline (norepinephrine) from a functioning third-order sympathetic neurone and so will dilate the pupil in first- or second-order lesions as well as the normal pupil. Adrenaline (epinephrine) 0.1% dilates the pupil of a third-order lesion due to denervation hypersensitivity.

39.
a. A feathery deep stromal scar and ghost vessels characteristic of interstitial keratitis.
b. The ghost vessels may refill and, rarely, bleed if the inflammation reactivates.
c. Bony features include sabre tibiae, saddle-shaped nose, frontal bossing, prognathism, high-arched palate, dental malformations (Hutchinson's teeth and Moon's molars) and sensorineural deafness.

40.

    a. The lens is subluxated upwards.

    b. Marfan's syndrome, associated with a mutation of the fibrillin gene on chromosome 15.

    c. Tall, but with arm span greater than height, muscular underdevelopment, hernias, aortic dilatation and dissection, heart valve disease, striae and fragility of the skin.

    d. Homocystinuria, Weill–Marchesani syndrome, hyperlysinaemia, sulphite oxidase deficiency, Ehlers–Danlos syndrome and Stickler's syndrome.

41.

    a. 90% or more of patients are positive for HLA-A29.

    b. Yes, moderate vitritis is typical.

    c. Electroretinography (ERG), which provides a baseline measure of retinal function.

    d. Optic atrophy and chronic cystoid macular oedema.

42.

    a. Arthritis (especially knees and ankles), plantar fasciitis, Achilles tendonitis, keratoderma blenorrhagica, mouth ulceration, balanitis, epididymitis, orchitis and prostatitis.

    b. Acute anterior uveitis and occasionally punctate epithelial keratitis.

    c. HLA-typing will be positive for HLA-B27 in 70% of cases.

    d. Aortic incompetence.

43.

    a. Ocular discomfort, double vision, reduced vision and cosmetic problems.

    b. The incidence is far higher in hyperthyroidism (thyrotoxicosis) than hypothyroidism (myxoedema). However, patients can be clinically and biochemically euthyroid.

    c. Failure of adduction.

    d. Systemic steroids, orbital radiotherapy and surgical decompression.

44.

    a. Recurrent, non-scarring blisters and sparse localized erythematous plaques.

    b. Symblepharon (adhesions between bulbar and palpebral conjunctiva), ankyloblepharon (adhesions between the lids at the outer canthus) and severe dry eye. Advanced disease can involve severe secondary corneal changes, which may cause blindness.

    c. Topical lubricants, steroids and antibiotics where appropriate; subconjunctival mitomycin C; protective contact lenses; systemic options include steroids, dapsone, intravenous immunoglobulins and cytotoxic agents.

45.

    a. Idiopathic intracranial hypertension, although CT or MRI brain scan is required to rule out a space-occupying lesion.

    b. Blindness may result from secondary optic atrophy due to chronic papilloedema.

    c. Diuretics, systemic steroids, optic nerve fenestration and lumboperitoneal shunt.

46. *a.* In pure graft failure, which occurs because of endothelial decompensation, the eye is quiet, whereas rejection involves an inflammatory element (although this may be mild). Specific signs of epithelial (discrete subepithelial infiltrates – Krachmer's spots) or endothelial (keratic precipitates, oedema, more marked inflammation) rejection will be evident. Failure is often a consequence of rejection.

   b. The mainstay of treatment is topical steroids, although periocular injection or systemic immunosuppression may be necessary.

   c. Eyelid disease, tear film dysfunction, anterior segment inflammation, corneal vascularization or thinning and uncontrolled glaucoma.

47. *a.* A pterygium, an area of degenerative fibrovascular tissue encroaching on the cornea most commonly seen in hot, dry climates.

   b. Visual deterioration (due to astigmatism or visual axis obstruction), substantial irritation and cosmesis.

   c. Simple removal is associated with a high rate of recurrence. Conjunctival patch autografting, irradiation and antimitotic agent application are more effective.

48. *a.* Choroidal folds.

   b. Idiopathic, because of bilateral involvement, lack of symptoms and the presence of hypermetropia.

   c. Orbital disease (e.g. thyroid, tumours) and ocular causes (e.g. hypotony, choroidal tumours, posterior scleritis, chronic papilloedema and scleral buckling).

49. *a.* No. The defects involve the temporal field of each eye; by definition, a bitemporal hemianopia.

   b. Chiasmal compression by a space-occupying lesion such as a pituitary adenoma needs to be excluded urgently. 'Tilted' optic discs, relatively common in myopes, can also give a similar field pattern, although the defects typically cross the midline.

   c. MRI of the brain and orbits, to include the optic chiasm.

50. *a.* The hands show features typical of rheumatoid arthritis.

   b. She almost certainly has dry eyes: keratoconjunctivitis sicca, i.e. secondary Sjögren's syndrome.

   c. Slit-lamp assessment of the tear film may show debris, froth, an irregular or thin marginal meniscus and a short break-up time. Other tests include staining the cornea and conjunctiva with rose Bengal and fluorescein, and the Schirmer test.

   d. Keratitis (which can be severe, with melting and perforation), and scleritis. Acquired Brown's syndrome is very rare.

51. *a.* A right lower motor neurone facial nerve palsy.

   b. Exposure keratopathy secondary to poor eyelid closure; cosmetic implications may also be substantial.

c. Topical lubricants may suffice in mild cases. Botulinum-induced ptosis is useful in recovering palsies but surgery will be necessary for profound permanent deficit (e.g. tarsorrhaphy, lid shortening and nerve grafting).

52.
a. Probably not, as the optic discs appear normal.
b. Approximately 10% at 5 years.
c. If the disc is unusually small, the physiological cup size might be considerably smaller than that shown.
d. Visual fields, to exclude glaucomatous changes and act as a baseline for monitoring purposes; pachymetry for central corneal thickness, as the measured intraocular pressure is higher than the true level in eyes with thick corneas; and baseline optic disc imaging, preferably with computed parameter analysis.

53.
a. Corneal calcium deposition in an interpalpebral distribution (band keratopathy).
b. Some children with JIA develop a chronic anterior uveitis, which can lead to secondary glaucoma, band keratopathy and cataract. The eye typically remains white and comfortable despite active inflammation so that the diagnosis may be overlooked.
c. Early-onset pauciarticular disease, the presence of serum antinuclear antibodies, and HLA-DR5 positivity.

54.
a. Contact lens-related keratitis, which clinically appears to be bacterial.
b. Corneal scraping for microscopy, culture and antibiotic sensitivity testing, followed by intensive topical broad-spectrum antibiotics. Admission to hospital is usually advisable. A mydriatic may improve comfort and prevent posterior synechiae formation. Oral antibiotics are sometimes used for ulcers near the limbus.
c. Acanthamoeba, fungi, atypical mycobacteria and herpes simplex.

55.
a. Right internuclear ophthalmoplegia (INO).
b. The right medial longitudinal fasciculus (MLF); the side of the lesion in the MLF corresponds to the eye that fails to adduct (the right eye in 55a).
c. Multiple sclerosis.
d. Stroke, tumours, trauma, encephalitis, drugs and hydrocephalus.

56.
a. Acute retinal necrosis; in this age group, varicella is the likely cause.
b. Polymerase chain reaction (PCR) analysis of aqueous and vitreous for viral DNA.
c. Intravenous aciclovir for 10 days then orally for 3 months; systemic steroids 24 hours after commencement of antiviral therapy.

57.
a. Rubeosis iridis, which develops in about 50% of ischaemic CRVOs and often results in neovascular glaucoma.

b. Diabetes, central retinal artery occlusion, carotid obstructive disease and chronic intraocular inflammation.

c. Urgent panretinal photocoagulation. If this fails to induce regression prior to irreversible pressure elevation, cyclodiode laser or drainage surgery can be carried out. The visual prognosis is very poor.

58.

a. The cornea is cloudy the anterior chamber shallow and the pupil dilated. The diagnosis is acute angle-closure glaucoma, in which the abdominal symptoms may occasionally be so severe as to constitute the main focus. Intraocular pressure measurement will confirm the diagnosis.

b. Admission to hospital, intravenous acetazolamide and topical agents to lower the intraocular pressure, followed by laser iridotomy to both eyes.

c. Acute iritis, corneal abrasion, keratitis and scleritis.

59.

a. Capillary haemangioma or 'strawberry naevus'.

b. Yes, because the lesion may induce amblyopia as a result of associated ptosis or strabismus.

c. Intralesional steroid injection. However, most strawberry naevi constitute only a cosmetic problem and can be left alone in anticipation of spontaneous resolution by the age of 7 years.

d. Very rarely, capillary haemangioma is part of a wider syndrome – Maffucci's (multiple systemic haemangiomata and bone lesions) or Kasabach–Merritt (haematological abnormalities).

60.

a. Levator palpebrae superioris and Müller's muscle; the former is supplied by the superior division of the oculomotor nerve and the latter by the sympathetic component of the autonomic nervous system.

b. • *Neurogenic*: third nerve palsy, Horner's syndrome, Marcus Gunn's ('jaw-winking') syndrome.
   • *Aponeurotic*: involutional (age-related), postoperative.
   • *Mechanical*: oedema, tumours, heavy redundant skin, cicatricial.
   • *Myogenic*: simple congenital, blepharophimosis syndrome, myasthenia gravis, ocular myopathy, myotonic dystrophy.

c. • *Proptosis of the contralateral eye*
   • *Eyelid*: redundant skin overhanging lid margin (dermatochalasis)
   • *Globe*: microphthalmos, phthisis
   • *Eye muscles*: vertical muscle imbalance
   • *Orbit*: enophthalmos.

61.

a. A limbal dermoid.

b. A choristoma, a congenital growth of normal tissue at an abnormal location.

c. For visual interference, irritation, or cosmesis.

d. Limbal dermoids are usually an isolated abnormality but may on occasion be part of Goldenhar's syndrome, Treacher Collins' syndrome or the naevus sebaceous syndrome of Jadassohn.

62.

a. Failure of elevation of the left eye in adduction, consistent with a left Brown's syndrome.

b. As with all squints, refraction, media and fundus examination and treatment of amblyopia are important. Surgery is needed only if there is significant deviation in the primary position, diplopia or an anomalous head posture.

c. Inflammation (e.g. rheumatoid arthritis), trauma and superior oblique surgery.

63.

a. Giant cell arteritis should be suspected and enquiry made concerning headache, scalp tenderness, jaw claudication, muscle girdle (particularly neck) aching, malaise, loss of weight and specifically previous diagnosis of polymyalgia rheumatica.

b. Erythrocyte sedimentation rate (ESR) and C-reactive protein (CRP); however, the diagnosis is not excluded by a low result nor categorically confirmed by a high one.

c. Temporal artery biopsy. Systemic (usually intravenous) steroids must be commenced immediately in this situation and should not be delayed while biopsy is awaited.

64.

a. Kearns–Sayre syndrome, which is characterized by pigmentary retinopathy and chronic progressive external ophthalmoplegia. The child may also have ataxia, deafness, diabetes and other systemic abnormalities.

b. Mitochondrial DNA deletions.

c. ECG shows cardiac conduction defects, CSF is abnormal and muscle biopsy shows the 'ragged red fibre' pattern.

65.

a. Iridoschisis, a very rare gradual splitting of the iris into anterior and posterior lamellae with disintegration of the anterior layer.

b. IOP elevation. It is postulated that episodic angle-closure glaucoma associated with very high IOP leads to the iris changes, rather than the iris changes precipitating the initiating event.

c. Laser peripheral iridotomy, followed by medical treatment as appropriate.

66.

a. Stenosis of the lower eyelid punctum. There is also a degree of medial ectropion resulting in the punctum pointing away from the lacus lacrimalis.

b. Further assessment falls into two categories: exclusion of any cause of ocular irritation, particularly 'paradoxical' lacrimation due to dry eye, and obstruction elsewhere in the lacrimal drainage system. Basic assessment of the lacrimal canaliculi and nasolacrimal duct involves syringing with saline.

c. Simple dilation of the punctum or incisional ('one-' or 'two-snip') enlargement of the canaliculus, combined if necessary with ectropion repair.

67.
a. The right cornea is larger than the left, although the left also appears enlarged. The most likely diagnosis is primary congenital glaucoma, although other causes of large corneas, large eyes and secondary infantile glaucoma must be excluded.
b. Breaks in Descemet's membrane ('Haab striae' when healed), an abnormal anterior chamber angle and optic disc cupping.
c. Examination under general anaesthesia will be necessary to facilitate gonioscopy, measurement of intraocular pressure and corneal diameter.

68.
a. Marginal keratitis.
b. It is not always possible to be certain but the overall clinical picture should be considered. Important points include: the relatively mild symptoms, the absence of predisposing factors such as contact lens wear, the distribution of the infiltrate in a band parallel to the limbus but separated by a clear zone. Typically the infiltrate is much larger than any associated epithelial defect. Chronic anterior blepharitis is often present.
c. A short course of weak topical steroid (e.g. fluorometholone).

69.
a. A hyphaema, a common complication of moderate to severe blunt trauma; blood in the anterior chamber which has settled to form a 'fluid level'.
b. The major risk is of a further bleed with resultant elevation of intraocular pressure, which can potentially lead to permanent corneal bloodstaining. Possible damage to anterior and posterior segment structures must also be assessed.
c. Activity is severely restricted, sometimes with hospital admission. The patient is initially reviewed daily. Other measures may include immobilization of the pupil with atropine, administration of an oral antifibrinolytic agent and treatment of anterior uveitis or raised pressure.

70.
a. A corneal abrasion.
b. Typically, the symptoms of an abrasion are severe: marked grittiness, redness, lacrimation and photophobia. Spontaneous recurrence of the epithelial defect is common (recurrent erosion syndrome).
c. Antibiotic ointment, cycloplegia to reduce discomfort, and oral analgesia; firm padding of the eye may improve comfort in a large abrasion but probably does not speed resolution. A bandage contact lens is sometimes used.

71.
a. Isolated left third (oculomotor) cranial nerve palsy.
b. A compressive lesion, particularly posterior communicating artery aneurysm.
c. Clinical features increasing the level of suspicion of a compressive lesion include pupillary involvement, headache or ocular pain,

younger patient age and absence of known vascular risk factors such as diabetes. A careful history and examination for additional neurological features is essential, followed by CNS imaging if appropriate. There is a wide range of causes of third nerve palsy; 25% are idiopathic.

72. *a.* Proliferative vitreoretinopathy (PVR).
b. Vitreous haze and condensation; pigment cells on the inferior retina; rolling of the edges of retinal breaks; wrinkling of the inner retinal surface; full-thickness retinal folds; subretinal strands.
c. Pars plana vitrectomy, if necessary using silicone oil tamponade and peeling, segmentation or delamination of epiretinal membranes.

73. *a.* Vitreous haemorrhage.
b. B-scan ultrasonography, principally to exclude retinal detachment.
c. Examples include proliferative retinopathies (diabetic, retinal vein occlusion, Eales's disease, retinopathy of prematurity, sickle-cell disease), posterior vitreous detachment and retinal tears, 'breakthrough' bleeding from choroidal neovascularization, and trauma.

74. *a.* A macular epiretinal membrane. A dense membrane is usually referred to as 'macular pucker' and a thinner membrane as in 'cellophane maculopathy'.
b. Membranes consist of retinal glial cells proliferating at the vitreoretinal interface, having reached the retinal surface via breaks in the internal limiting membrane.
c. Retinal surgery and photocoagulation, trauma, inflammation and retinal vascular disease.

75. *a.* Infusion cannula (lower right), light pipe and vitreous cutter.
b. • Rhegmatogenous retinal detachment associated with the following: significant PVR, media opacity precluding adequate retinal view (vitreous haemorrhage, posterior lens capsular opacity), giant retinal tears and posterior breaks including macular holes.
• Tractional retinal detachment, usually diabetic or traumatic.
• Persistent vitreous haemorrhage.
• Removal of intraocular foreign body.
• Severe endophthalmitis.
• Age-related macular hole.
• Macular degeneration: excision of choroidal neovascular membranes, macular translocation.

76. *a.* With recurrent erosions at the end of the first decade.
b. Irregular bands of collagen, staining blue with Masson trichrome, replace the Bowman layer which may even be absent.
c. Autosomal dominant; the gene is located at 10q24.

d. Reis–Bücklers dystrophy (Bowman layer type 1), in which the honeycomb pattern assumed by the opacities is considerably less prominent.

77.
a. Normal right abduction but limited left abduction associated with retraction of the globe and narrowing of the palpebral fissure. The diagnosis is left Duane's retraction syndrome.
b. This patient can be classified as Huber type 1:
   • Huber type 1: limited abduction
   • Huber type 2: limited adduction
   • Huber type 3: limited abduction and adduction.
c. Anisometropia, coloboma, microphthalmos and heterochromia.

78.
a. The disc is enlarged and is surrounded by a hypopigmented ring. The emerging blood vessels manifest a radial pattern. The excavation is funnel-shaped and contains a central core of whitish glial tissue. The diagnosis is morning glory anomaly.
b. Approximately 30%.
c. These are uncommon: frontonasal dysplasia, which includes facial and midline neurological abnormalities, and neurofibromatosis type 2.

79.
a. Computed corneal topographic imaging: 'corneal topography' or mapping.
b. The contour of the cornea at differing locations; colours at the red end of the scale are used to represent steep corneal regions, with the flattest areas shown as blue.
c. The contours demonstrated are consistent with keratoconus. In the right eye the cone is located inferiorly with dioptric values at the apex reaching 56 D; in the left the cone is central with values up to 63 D.

80.
a. Myasthenia gravis.
b. Fatigue on sustained upgaze with worsening of ptosis. Cogan's lid twitch – overshoot on moving from depression to primary position in myasthenia. Ice test – reduced ptosis after ice pack applied for 2 minutes.
c. Acetylcholine receptor antibody levels.
d. Edrophonium (an anticholinesterase) testing: significant temporary improvement in ptosis and/or diplopia following intravenous administration.

81.
a. A keratoprosthesis or artificial corneal implant.
b. When the cornea is severely damaged but the retina and optic nerve retain good function and conventional corneal grafting has an extremely poor prognosis.
c. Endophthalmitis, glaucoma, retroprosthesis membrane formation and extrusion.

82.   *a.* Right cataract and heterochromia iridis. These findings, together with
      the stellate keratic precipitates, suggest Fuchs' uveitis syndrome.
   b. Glaucoma, and occasionally severe vitreous opacities.
   c. Topical steroids are not beneficial and may promote glaucoma and
      cataract. Severe vitreous opacities may benefit from periocular steroid
      injection.

83.   *a.* Significant posterior capsular opacification.
   b. Glare.
   c. Nd:YAG laser capsulotomy.
   d. Retinal detachment, cystoid macular oedema, lens dislocation,
      intraocular pressure elevation (usually transient) and visually
      inconsequential pitting of the implant.

84.   *a.* A lower lid entropion.
   b. Age-related horizontal lid laxity, weakening of the effect of the lower
      lid retractors and over-riding of the pretarsal by the preseptal
      orbicularis oculi with associated prolapse of orbital fat.
   c. Surgical options depend on the presence or absence of horizontal lid
      laxity and include simple everting sutures, the horizontal lid-splitting
      Wies procedure, inferior retractor tightening (Jones procedure) and
      horizontal lid shortening.

85.   *a.* Numerous large drusen.
   b. Fundus fluorescein angiography would demonstrate CNV and aid in
      deciding whether treatment is indicated and what form this should
      take.
   c. A specific antioxidant vitamin and mineral supplement regimen
      reduces the risk of CNV in patients fitting certain criteria, including
      the situation described.

86.   *a.* Indocyanine green angiography (ICG); the wavelengths used penetrate
      blood and pigment more effectively than fluorescein angiography and
      ICG is therefore superior for investigating retinal pathology in some
      circumstances.
   b. This is a late phase ICG of a pigment epithelial detachment (PED).
   c. A thickened degenerate Bruch membrane may impede the transit of
      fluid from the retinal pigment epithelium (RPE) to the choroid.
   d. There is no treatment for PEDs; laser photocoagulation may cause
      tearing of the RPE. Spontaneous resolution sometimes occurs.

87.   *a.* Several large haemorrhages with white centres (Roth spots) which
      usually represent fibrin emboli occluding ruptured blood vessels.
   b. This patient requires urgent investigation. Other causes include
      anaemia, bacterial endocarditis, diabetes and dysproteinaemia.
   c. Other fundus changes include cotton wool spots, haemorrhages,
      peripheral retinal neovascularization, a 'leopard spot' fundus and

infiltration of the optic nerve head. Elsewhere in the eye, subconjunctival haemorrhage, orbital involvement, iritis, pseudohypopyon and hyphaema may occur.

88.
a. Given the marked iris transillumination and the extremely pale skin and hair, tyrosinase-negative.

b. Patients with tyrosinase-negative oculocutaneous albinism have a decreased number of crossing nerve fibres at the optic chiasm, as well as other central visual pathway anomalies.

c. Chediak–Higashi syndrome (white-cell-related immunodeficiency) and Hermansky–Pudlak syndrome (a lysosomal storage disease with platelet dysfunction).

d. No, because only tyrosinase-positive albinism is associated with these syndromes.

89.
a. An area of chorioretinal atrophy associated with retinal pigment epithelial hyperplasia. The most common cause of this appearance is old congenital toxoplasmosis.

b. Usually in the teens to thirties. In the immunocompromised, however, reactivation of congenitally acquired infection or acquisition of new infection commonly occurs at any age.

c. Serology for toxoplasma antibodies but the titre, however, does not correlate with activity. Polymerase chain reaction (PCR) DNA testing of a vitreous biopsy sample may be diagnostic.

90.
a. A fluorescein angiogram showing the petalloid hyperfluorescent pattern characteristic of cystoid macular oedema.

b. The prolapse of vitreous gel into the anterior segment from its physiological location in the posterior segment, usually by inadvertent rupture of the posterior capsule or zonules.

c. Increased risk of cystoid macular oedema, retinal detachment, endophthalmitis, uveitis, glaucoma, corneal decompensation and lens implant dislocation.

91.
a. A silicone explant, placed during the surgery, has eroded through the conjunctiva.

b. At this stage, it should be safe to remove the explant without precipitating re-detachment. Removal in the first few months, however, carries a 5–10% risk.

c. Under sterile conditions: if very loose, the explant can simply be lifted gently out of its position and any visible sutures trimmed; if firmly attached, conjunctival dissection and suture release is necessary.

92.
a. Large ('mutton fat') keratic precipitates characteristic of granulomatous uveitis.

b. Yes. Granulomatous uveitis should always be investigated, except in the presence of a previously established systemic illness.

c. Where appropriate, initial screening might include a full blood count, ESR, serum angiotensin-converting enzyme, syphilis serology and chest X-ray (e.g. tuberculosis, sarcoidosis).

93.
a. Osteogenesis imperfecta. Types 1 and 2 are associated with blue sclera.
b. The blue appearance is caused by a collagen abnormality leading to relative scleral transparency.
c. The more important include Ehlers–Danlos syndrome (usually type 6, although blue sclera has been reported in other types), pseudoxanthoma elasticum (dominant type 2), and Turner's syndrome.

94.
a. Extensive chorioretinal atrophy, a form of myopic maculopathy.
b. Other macular changes include choroidal neovascularization (CNV), haemorrhage without CNV, lacquer cracks (which predispose to CNV), macular hole and pigment proliferation (Fuchs spot). Highly myopic eyes have a predisposition to retinal detachment, cataract and glaucoma.
c. Nearer 30 mm.

95.
a. Laser in-situ keratomileusis (LASIK), in which a hinged flap as shown is cut from the corneal surface, excimer laser ablation is performed on the exposed stroma and the flap is replaced.
b. Yes, but only to a limited extent: approximately 4 D of hypermetropia and 5 D of astigmatism.
c. Operative buttonholing of the flap and corneal perforation; postoperative infection, sterile diffuse lamellar keratitis (DLK or 'sands of the Sahara'), flap dislocation or wrinkling, persistent epithelial defects and epithelial ingrowth under the flap.

96.
a. Episcleritis (strictly simple sectorial episcleritis, the commonest type).
b. Simple or nodular; the former may be sectorial or diffuse.
c. In contrast to scleritis, systemic investigation is not appropriate because the prevalence of an associated systemic disease is extremely low.
d. Mild cases are self-limiting and require no treatment. Topical steroids or oral non-steroidal anti-inflammatory drugs are sometimes needed in severe or persistent cases.

97.
a. A spontaneous subconjunctival haemorrhage (SCH).
b. Mild discomfort.
c. Blood pressure should be checked, because spontaneous SCH is twice as common in patients with hypertension as those without. No further investigation is necessary, even if bleeding should recur at the same site. If both eyes are involved or there is other cause for suspicion of a bleeding diathesis, further assessment might be considered.

98.
  a. A localized detachment of the neurosensory retina at the macula – central serous retinopathy.
  b. Approximately 6/12, characteristically improved by a weak 'plus' (convex) lens.
  c. Fundus fluorescein angiography will usually demonstrate an 'ink-blot' or 'smoke-stack' pattern of increasing hyperfluorescence.

99.
  a. Intermittent exotropia.
  b. Basic exotropia, in which the angle is the same for near and distance; convergence weakness, where the deviation is greater for near; divergence excess, with a greater deviation for distance.
  c. As with all squints, media and fundus examination followed by refraction is the initial step. Spectacle correction of myopia may stimulate accommodation such that the squint is controlled. Orthoptic treatment is sometimes effective but surgery is frequently necessary.

100.
  a. Defective visual acuity persisting after correction of refractive error and removal of visual pathway pathology, if present.
  b. Amblyopia commonly occurs in association with strabismus, when the image from the deviating eye is suppressed by the brain during the critical developmental period. It can also be caused by anisometropia (difference in refraction between the eyes), stimulus deprivation (cataract) and ametropia (bilateral high refractive error).
  c. This varies according to parent and child motivation and other factors, but is probably around 7–8 years in strabismic amblyopia and up to 12 years for anisometropic.

101.
  a. A Kayser–Fleischer ring.
  b. Deposition of copper granules in the peripheral region of Descemet's membrane.
  c. Wilson's disease, an abnormality of copper metabolism caused by a deficiency of caeruloplasmin.
  d. Anterior capsular 'sunflower' cataract.
  e. Liver disease and basal ganglia dysfunction

102.
  a. The cornea shows a branching, whorled pattern with its centre located inferior to the pupil, consisting of very fine deposits within the epithelium: vortex keratopathy or cornea verticillata.
  b. Amiodarone.
  c. Virtually all patients receiving amiodarone develop corneal changes.
  d. Other drugs include chloroquine and hydroxychloroquine. Fabry's disease, a glycolipidosis, is also associated with vortex keratopathy.

103.
  a. No. Keratoconus is extremely unlikely to present at this age.
  b. Involvement specifically of the peripheral rather than central cornea leads the ophthalmologist towards a number of defined conditions having a predilection for this site.

c. Taking account of the patient's gender, absence of known systemic disease, absence of inflammation, involvement of both eyes and the appearance of the cornea, this is likely to be Terrien's marginal degeneration. This condition is an uncommon idiopathic painless thinning of the peripheral cornea; the main visual effect is astigmatism.

104.
a. Axial proptosis.
b. Cavernous haemangioma. 70% of these occur in women and the majority are located within the muscle cone.
c. Optic disc swelling or pallor, choroidal folds and ocular motility disturbance.
d. Surgical excision; the tumour is usually well encapsulated.

105.
a. B-scan ultrasonography, which produces a two-dimensional section of the tissue scanned. A-scan ultrasonography produces a one-dimensional scan and is principally used in biometric calculation of intraocular lens implant power.
b. A hyperdense signal is evident at the optic nerve head, consistent with optic disc drusen, a cause of pseudopapilloedema.
c. Fluorescein angiography will demonstrate autofluorescence of superficial disc drusen and absence of leakage that would occur in true disc swelling. CT scanning will show any calcification of the drusen.

106.
a. Progressive iris atrophy, a variant of iridocorneal endothelial (ICE) syndrome, characterized by a proliferation of abnormal corneal endothelial cells across the anterior chamber angle and iris.
b. Iris naevus (Cogan–Reese) syndrome, characterized by a diffuse iris naevus with associated iris atrophy in about 50% of cases, and Chandler's syndrome, in which corneal changes predominate.
c. Approximately 50%.

107.
a. A displaced pupil (corectopia), full-thickness iris defects (pseudopolycoria) and cataract.
b. Rieger's syndrome, a variant of the Axenfeld–Rieger syndrome.
c. Inheritance is autosomal dominant; genes implicated include *FOXC1* on chromosome 6p25, and *PITX2* on chromosome 4q25.
d. About 50%, usually during childhood or early adulthood.

108.
a. A large hypopyon.
b. Bacterial endophthalmitis.
c. Initially, vitreous biopsy and intravitreal antibiotics. The benefit of topical, periocular injection and systemic antibiotics is not clear, but are often used. Systemic steroids are often given to reduce inflammation. Vitrectomy is of benefit only if vision is reduced to 'light perception'.

109. *a.* A Krukenberg spindle.
   b. Pigment dispersion syndrome.
   c. Most patients with this condition are myopic.
   d. Up to 50% of patients may eventually develop glaucoma.

110. *a.* Thickening, reddening and telangiectasia of the lid margin skin, with crusting and scaling around the lashes, particularly at the bases.
   b. This patient has anterior blepharitis, predominantly of the staphylococcal type.
   c. An approximate ascending hierarchy of treatment: rigorous daily lid hygiene regimen, topical lubricants, lid margin antibiotic ointment, intermittent systemic antibiotics (e.g. tetracycline, doxycycline) and weak topical steroids.

111. *a.* A corneoscleral penetrating injury with a flat anterior chamber.
   b. Ideally, CT scanning should be carried out to exclude an intraocular or intraorbital foreign body. Primary wound repair should be undertaken within a few hours with the intention of restoring the integrity of the eye wall and preventing infection; a careful search for occult wounds should be carried out as part of the procedure. Antibiotics are administered as appropriate. It should be remembered that systemic stabilization and management of any life-threatening injuries has priority.

112. *a.* Nd:YAG (neodymium: yttrium–aluminium–garnet) iridotomy.
   b. A sudden and severe spike in intraocular pressure sufficient to cause corneal oedema can be caused by intermittent subacute primary angle-closure (including plateau iris syndrome), Posner–Schlossmann syndrome, pigment dispersion syndrome, herpetic keratouveitis and occasionally pseudoexfoliative glaucoma.
   c. Capsulotomy, disruption of vitreous strands in the anterior chamber and disruption of the posterior hyaloid face to disperse premacular blood.

113. *a.* Lattice dystrophy type 3 or 3a; the former is probably of autosomal recessive inheritance and the latter autosomal dominant.
   b. No.
   c. This is necessary in most cases to improve vision.
   d. Type 1 (Biber–Haab–Dimmer), which presents in the first decade with recurrent erosions, and Type 2 (Meretoja's syndrome), a systemic amyloidosis that presents in middle age with facial palsy and corneal involvement.

114. *a.* Retinopathy of prematurity.
   b. Stage 1: Demarcation line at the border of vascularized and avascular retina
      Stage 2: Ridge at the same site

Stage 3: Extraretinal fibrovascular proliferation (shown in the illustration)

Stage 4: Subtotal retinal detachment

Stage 5: Total retinal detachment

Plus disease: Posterior pole vascular engorgement, vitreous haze, poor mydriasis.

 c. Threshold disease, consisting of five contiguous or eight non-contiguous clock-hours of stage 3 together with 'plus' disease. Surgery may be carried out for stage 4 or 5.

 d. Laser or cryotherapy to the avascular area.

115. a. Measurement of the blood pressure because the signs are highly suggestive of severe hypertensive retinopathy.

 b. Because the deposits are located in the retinal layer of Henle and follow the fibre arrangement accordingly.

 c. Exudative retinal detachment (particularly in toxaemia of pregnancy), Elschnig spots (focal choroidal infarcts), and Siegrist streaks, (flecks along choroidal vessels indicating fibrinoid necrosis).

116. a. Lisch nodules.

 b. Neurofibromatosis-1.

 c. Eyelid neurofibroma, glaucoma, optic nerve glioma, ectropion uveae, prominent corneal nerves, choroidal naevi and melanomas, retinal astrocytomas, and spheno-orbital encephalocele.

 d. Autosomal dominant with irregular penetrance and variable expressivity; the gene locus is on chromosome 17q11.

117. a. A printout of frequency-doubling perimetry (commonly referred to as frequency-doubling technology, FDT).

 b. FDT specifically targets the magnocellular ganglion cells, which are damaged early on in the course of glaucoma. It does this by utilizing the illusion of frequency doubling produced by a low spatial frequency grating undergoing high temporal frequency reversal.

 c. It is much quicker and easier to perform than conventional automated perimetry.

118. a. Salzmann's nodular degeneration.

 b. Trachoma is the likely cause in this patient.

 c. Often, no treatment is required. If the eyes are irritable, topical lubricants can be used. Superficial keratectomy or lamellar keratoplasty may be necessary in severe cases.

119. a. A chalazion, which is caused by a granulomatous inflammatory reaction to accumulated secretions in a blocked meibomian gland.

 b. A conjunctival granuloma.

 c. Chalazia may resolve spontaneously. Persistent lesions are usually treated by curettage and, rarely, by local steroid injection. Topical or systemic antibiotics may be required for an acutely inflamed or infected lesion.

120. *a.* Myelinated nerve fibres.

b. An enlarged blind spot may be present with a peripapillary lesion, and peripheral lesions may give corresponding field defects. Myopia and amblyopia may be associated, and symptomatic macular involvement has been reported. Rarely, associated retinal vascular abnormalities can be present.

c. Myelinated fibres may represent a choristoma resulting from ectopic oligodendrocytes.

d. About 1%.

Index

Page numbers in *italics* refer to questions and corresponding answes

A

Abducens nerve palsy, 88. 89
Abrasion, corneal, 90, 91, *122, 158*
Acanthamoeba keratitis, 28, 29
Acetazolamide, *156*
Acquired maculopathies, 72–73
Actinic keratosis, 8, 9
Acute allergic conjunctivitis, 20, 21
Acute multifocal posterior placoid pigment epitheliopathy (AMPPPE), 48, 49, *99, 148*
Adenoma sebaceum, *98, 148*
Adenoviral conjunctivitis, 20, 21
Age-related macular degeneration, 70–71, *106:151, 128:161*
AIDS, molluscum contagiosum in, 4, *4, 102, 149*
Albinism, *129, 162*
Amaurosis fugax, 66
Amblyopia, 86, *135, 164*
Amiodarone, corneal deposits in, *136, 164*
Angioid streaks, 72, 73, *100, 148–149*
Angle-recession glaucoma, 52, 53
Aniridia, 58, 59, *92, 145*
Ankyloblepharon, 26, *153*
Antioxidants, 70, *128, 161*
Antiviral agents, 30, 32, *105:151, 115:155*
Artificial corneal implant (keratoprosthesis), *126, 160*
Astigmatism
    correction, *132, 163*
Astrocytoma, retinal, 80, 81, *98, 148*
Atopic keratoconjunctivitis, 22
Axenfeld–Rieger syndrome, 58, 59, *138, 165*

B

Bacterial conjunctivitis, 20, 21
Bacterial endophthalmitis, 60, *139, 165*
Bacterial keratitis, 28, 29
Band keratopathy, 42, 43, *114, 155*
Basal cell carcinoma, 8, 9, *92, 145*

Basal cell papilloma, 6, 7
Behçet's disease, 46, 47, *103, 150*
Best's disease, 74, 75
Biber–Haab–Dimmer degeneration, *141, 166*
Bielschowsky test, 88, 89
Birdshot retinochoroidopathy, 48, 49, *109, 153*
Blepharitis, 2–3, *140, 166*
Blepharophimosis syndrome, 10, 11
Blow-out fracture, 18, 19, *100, 148*
Blue sclera, *131, 163*
Blunt trauma, 90, 91, *121, 158*
Bournville's disease, 80, *98, 148*
Bowman layer dystrophies, 34, 35, *124, 159–160*
Brown's syndrome, 86, 87, *112:154, 118:157*
Bull's eye maculopathy, 72, 73
Buphthalmos, 58, 59

C

Candidal keratitis, 28
'Candlewax drippings', 46, 47
Capillary haemangioma
    eyelid, 6, 7, *117, 156*
    orbit, 16, 17
    retina, 80, 81, *94, 145–146*
Capsular opacification, 60, 61
Carotid-cavernous fistula, 18, 19
Cataract
    age-related, 60–61, *103, 150*
    infantile, 62, 63
    secondary, 62
Cataract surgery
    complications, *127:161, 130:162, 139:165*
    methods, 60, 61
Cavernous haemangioma
    orbit, 16, *137, 165*
    retina, 80, 81
Cellulitis, orbital, 18, 19, *97, 147*
Central serous retinopathy, *134, 164*
Chalazion (meibomian cyst), 4, 5, *144, 167–168*
Chandler's syndrome, *138, 165*
Chediak–Higashi syndrome, *129, 162*

Cherry-red spot, 66, 67, *107*, *151*
Chlamydial conjunctivitis, 20, 21, 22
Choristoma, conjunctival, 24, 25, *118*, *156*
Choroid
    detachment, *95*, *146*
    dystrophies, 74, 75
    folds, *112*, *154*
    haemangioma, 78, 79
    melanoma, 78, 79, *98*, *147–148*
    metastatic carcinoma, 78, 79
    naevus, 78, 79, *98*
    neovascularization (CNV), 70, 71,
        106:151, *128:161*
    osteoma, 78, 79
    rupture, 90, 91
Choroideremia, 74, 75
Choroidopathy, serpiginous, 48, 49
Cicatricial pemphigoid, 26, 27, *110*, *153*
Cicatrizing conjunctivitis, 26, 27
Clinically significant macular oedema
    (CSMO), 64, *98*, *147*
Cogan microcystic dystrophy, 34, 35
Cogan–Reese syndrome, *138*, *165*
Cogan's lid twitch, *126*, *160*
Collier's sign, *149*
Coloboma
    lens, 62, 63
    optic disc, 84, 85
Commotio retinae, 90, 91
Computed corneal topographic imaging,
        125, *160*
Congenital hypertrophy of the retinal
        pigment epithelium (CHRPE), *107*,
        152
Congenital syphilis, *108*, *152*
Conjunctival and corneal intra-epithelial
        neoplasia (CCIN), 24, 25
Conjunctival tumours, 24–25, *96:146*,
        118:156–157
Conjunctivitis
    acute, 20–21, *106*, *151*
    chronic, 22–23, *93*, *145*
    cicatrizing, 26, 27
Cornea
    abrasion, 90, 91, *122*, *158*
    dystrophies, 34–35, *124*, *159–160*
        epithelial basement membrane
            dystrophy, 34, 35
    foreign body trauma, 90, 91
    graft, 34, 35, *111*, *154*
    herpes simplex infection, 30–31, *105*,
        151
    implant, *126*, *160*
    pannus, 22, 23

    size and shape disorders, 38–39
    suppurative keratitis, 28–29, 114, 155
    topographic mapping, *125*, *160*
    ulceration, 36–37
    verticillata, *136*, *164*
Cotton-wool spots, 64, 65, 66, 69
'Cupid's bow' (pseudogerontoxon), 22, 23
Cyst of Moll, 4, 5
Cystoid macular oedema, *130*, *162*
Cyst of Zeis, 4, 5
Cytomegalovirus retinitis, 44, 45

D

Dacryocystorhinostomy, *95*, *146*
Dellen, corneal, 36, 37
Dermoid, limbal, 24, 25, *118*, *156*
Dermoid cyst, 16, 17
Diabetic maculopathy, 64, 65
Diabetic retinopathy, 64–65, *97:147*,
        98:147
Disciform keratitis, 30, 31
Distichiasis, 12
Drusen
    macular, 70, 71, *128*, *161*
    optic disc, 84, 85, *137*, *165*
Dry eye, 26, 27
Duane's syndrome, 86, 87, *124*, *160*

E

Ectopia lentis, 62, 63
Ectropion, 12, 13, *120*, *157*
Eczema of the eyelids, 3
Edrophonium test, *126*, *160*
Electroretinography, *153*
Elschnig spots, *167*
Entropion, 12, 13, *128*, *161*
Episcleritis, 40, 41, *133*, *163*
Esotropia, 86, 87, *104*, *150*
Exotropia, 86, 87, *134*, *164*
External hordeolum (stye), 4, 5
Exudative retinal detachment, 76, 77
Eyelid
    benign tumours, 6–7, *117*, *156*
    ectropion, 12, 13, *120*, *157*
    entropion, 12, 13, *128*, *161*
    non-neoplastic lumps, 4–5, *102:149*,
        144:168
    premalignant and malignant tumours,
        8–9, *92*, *145*
    see also Blepharitis; Ptosis

F

Fabry's disease, *136, 164*
Foreign body trauma, 90, 91
Fourth nerve palsy, 88, 89
Frequency-doubling technology (FDT), *143, 167*
Fuchs' endothelial dystrophy, 34, 35
Fuchs' spot, 72, 73
Fuchs' uveitis syndrome, 42, *127, 161*
Fundal dystrophies, 74–75, *107, 152*
Fundus flavimaculatus, 74, 75
Fungal keratitis, 28, 29

G

Giant cell arteritis, 82, *119, 157*
Giant papillary conjunctivitis, 22, 23, *93, 145*
Gillespie's syndrome, 58, *145*
Glaucoma
    angle-closure
        primary, 54–55, *116, 156*
        secondary, 56–57, *138, 165*
    congenital, 58, 59, *120, 158*
    developmental, 58–59, *120, 158*
    drainage device, 56, 57, *99, 148*
    neovascular, 56
    normal-tension, 50, *103:149-150, 112:154*
    open-angle
        pigmentary, 52, 53
        primary, 50–51, *93, 145*
        pseudoexfoliation, 52, 53, *94, 146*
        secondary, 52–53, *94:146, 139:166*
Glaukomflecken, 54, 55
Granular dystrophy, 34, 35
Granulomatous uveitis, 42, 43, *131, 162–163*
Grönblad–Strandberg syndrome, *100, 148*
Gyrate atrophy, 74, 75

H

Haab striae, 58, 59, *120, 158*
Haemangioma
    choroidal, 78, 79
    retinal, 80, 81, *94, 145–146*
    see also Capillary haemangioma;
        Cavernous haemangioma
Haemorrhage
    anterior chamber (hyphaema), 90, 91
    in hypertensive retinopathy, 68, 69
    retinal, in diabetic retinopathy, 64, 65
    in retinal vein occlusion, 66, 67
    spontaneous subconjunctival, *133, 163*
    vitreous, *123, 159*
Hay fever conjunctivitis, 20
Hering's law, *151*
Hermansky–Pudlak syndrome, *129, 162*
Herpes simplex infection, 20, 30–31, *105, 151*
Herpes zoster ophthalmicus, 32–33, *102:149, 115:155*
Hess chart, *106, 151*
Histoplasmosis, 44, 45
Horner's syndrome, 10, 11, *107, 152*
Hutchinson's sign, 32, *102, 149*
Hypermetropia correction, *132, 163*
Hypertensive retinopathy, 68, 69, *142, 167*
Hyphaema, 90, 91, *121, 158*

I

Ice test, *126, 160*
Idiopathic intracranial hypertension, *111, 153*
Idiopathic orbital inflammation
    (pseudotumour), 18, 19
Indocyanine green angiography, *128, 161*
Infantile cataract, 62, 63
Infective keratitis, 28–29, *114, 155*
Internal hordeolum (acute chalazion), 4, 5
Internuclear ophthalmoplegia, *115, 155*
Intraocular lens implant (IOL), 60, 61
Iridocorneal dysgenesis, 58, 59, *92, 145*
Iridocorneal endothelial (ICE) syndrome, 56, 57, *138, 165*
Iridodialysis, 90, 91
Iridoschisis, *119, 157*
Iris
    atrophy, 56, 57
    melanoma, 78, 79
    see also Aniridia
Iris naevus syndrome, *138, 165*
Iritis, 42, 56
Ischaemic central retinal vein occlusion, 66, 67, *116, 156*
Ischaemic optic neuropathy, 82, 83, *119, 157*

J

Juvenile idiopathic arthritis, 42, *114, 155*

K

Kasabach–Merritt syndrome, *117*, *156*
Kayser–Fleischer ring, *135*, *164*
Kearns–Sayre syndrome, *119*, *157*
Keratic precipitates, 42, 43, *131*, *162–163*
Keratitis
    contact lens-related, 28, 29, *114*, *155*
    fungal, 28, 29
    herpes simplex, 30–31, 105, 151
    herpes zoster, 32, 33, *102:149*
    interstitial, *108*, *152*
    marginal, 36, 37, *121*, *158*
    pseudomonas, 28, 29
    rosacea, 36, 37
    suppurative, 28–29, *114*, *155*
Keratoacanthoma, 6, 7
Keratoconjunctivitis
    atopic, 22
    sicca, 26, 27, *112*, *154*
    vernal, 22, 23
Keratoconus, 38, 39, *125:160*, *136:164–165*
Keratoglobus, 38, 39
Keratoprosthesis, *126*, *160*
Keratosis, actinic, 8, 9
Krukenberg spindle, 52, 53, *139*, *166*

L

Lacrimal system probing, *95*, *146*
Laser in-situ keratomileusis (LASIK), *132*,
    163
Lattice dystrophies, 34, 35, *141*, *166*
Lens disorders, 62–63
    see also Cataracts
Leukaemia, *129*, *161*
Leukocoria, 80, 81, *101*, *149*
Limbal dermoid, 24, 25, *118*, *156*
Lipodermoid, 24
Lisch nodules, *142*, *167*

M

Macular degeneration *see* Age-related
    macular degeneration
Macular epiretinal membrane, 72, 73, *123*,
    159
Macular hole, 72, 73, *104*, *150*
Macular oedema
    clinically significant, 64, *98*, *147*
    cystoid, *130*, *162*

Maculopathy
    acquired, 72–73, *100:149*, *104:150*,
        123:159, *132:163*
    diabetic, 64, 65
Maffucci's syndrome, *117*, *156*
Map–dot–fingerprint dystrophy, 34, 35
Marcus Gunn syndrome, 10, 11
Marfan's syndrome, 62, 63, *108*, *153*
Megalocornea, 38, 39
Meibomian gland
    cyst (chalazion), 4, 5, *144*, *167–168*
    dysfunction in blepharitis, 2, 3
Melanocytic naevus, 6, 7
Melanocytoma, optic nerve head, 80, 81
Melanoma
    choroidal, 78, 79, *98*, *147–148*
    conjunctival, 24, 25
    iris, 78, 79
Melanosis, conjunctival, 24, *96*, *146*
Meretoja's syndrome, *141*, *166*
Microcornea, 38, 39
Miller's syndrome, 58, *92*, *145*
Molluscum contagiosum, 4, 5, *102*, *149*
Mooren's ulcer, 36, 37
Morning glory anomaly, 84, 85, *125*, *160*
Multiple sclerosis, 82, *96:146–147*,
    115.155
Munson sign, 38, 39
'Mutton fat' keratic precipitates, 42, *131*,
    163
Myasthenia gravis, 10, *126*, *160*
Myelinated nerve fibres, *144*, *168*
Myopia correction, *132*, *163*
Myopic maculopathy, 72, 73, *132*, *163*
Myotonic dystrophy, ptosis, 11

N

Naevus
    choroidal, 78, 79, *98*
    conjunctival, 24, 25
    melanocytic, 6, 7
Nasolacrimal duct, congenital obstruction,
    95, *146*
Nd:YAG iridotomy, *141*, *166*
Neonatal conjunctivitis, 20, 21, *106*, *151*
Neovascular glaucoma, 56
Nerve palsies, 88–89, *106:151*, *113:155*,
    122:158–159
Neural tumours, 16, 17
Neurofibromatosis-1, 58, *142*, *167*
Nuclear sclerosis, 60, 61
Nystagmus, *115*, *155*

O

Oculocutaneous albinism, *129, 162*
Oculomotor nerve palsy, 88, 89, *122, 158–159*
Optic atrophy, 82, 83
Optic disc
    congenital anomalies, 84–85, *125, 160*
    normal, 51
Optic nerve glioma, 16
Optic nerve head
    drusen, 84, 85, *137, 165*
    infarction, 82, 83, *119, 157*
    melanocytoma, 80, 81
Optic nerve sheath meningioma, 16, 17
Optic neuritis, 82, 83, *96, 146–147*
Orbital cellulitis, 18, 19, *97, 147*
Orbital floor fracture, 18, 19, *100, 148*
Orbital pseudotumour, 18, 19
Orbital tumours, 16–17, *137, 165*
Orbital varices, 16, 17
Osteogenesis imperfecta, *131, 163*
Osteoma, choroidal, 78, 79

P

Papillary conjunctivitis, 22, 23
Papilloedema, 82, 83
Parinaud's (dorsal midbrain) syndrome, *101, 149*
Pars plana vitrectomy, 76, *123, 159*
Peau d'orange, *100, 149*
Penetrating keratoplasty (corneal graft), 34, 35, *111, 154*
Periphlebitis, 46, 47
Peters anomaly, 58
Phacomatoses, 58, 59, *94, 145–146*
Photodynamic therapy, 70
Phthisis bulbi, 42, 43
Pigmentary glaucoma, 52, 53
Pigment dispersion syndrome, 52, *139, 166*
Pigment epithelial detachment (PED), 70, *128, 161*
Pilocarpine, *156*
Pit, optic disc, 84, 85
Plexiform neurofibroma, 6, 7
Pneumococcal keratitis, 28, 29
Polypoidal choroidal vasculopathy (PCV), 70
Posterior lens capsular opacification, 60, 61, *127, 161*
Premature infants, retinopathy, 68, 69, *142, 167*

Primary acquired melanosis, 24, 25, *96, 146*
Primary congenital glaucoma, 58, 59, *120, 158*
Proliferative vitreoretinopathy, 76, 77, *123, 159*
Pseudoesotropia, 86, 87
Pseudoexanthoma elasticum, 72, *100, 148*
Pseudoexfoliative glaucoma, 52, 53, *94, 146*
Pseudogerontoxon, 22, 23
Pseudomonas keratitis, 28, 29
Pseudopapilloedema, 84, *137, 165*
Pseudoptosis, *117, 156*
Pseudotumour (idiopathic orbital inflammation), 18, 19
Pterygium, *111, 154*
Ptosis, 10–11, *117, 156*
Punctum
    stenosis of, *120, 157*

R

Racial epithelial melanosis, 24, *96, 146*
Recurrent erosion syndrome, 90, *122, 158*
Reis–Bücklers dystrophy, 34, *124, 160*
Reiter's syndrome, 42, *109, 153*
Retina
    acute necrosis, 32, *115, 155*
    astrocytoma, 80, 81, *98, 148*
    haemangioma, 80, 81, *94, 145–146*
    haemorrhages, *see* Haemorrhages, retina
    lattice degeneration, 76, 77
    retinoblastoma, 80, 81, *101, 149*
    tear formation, 90, *105, 150*
    trauma, 90, 91
Retinal artery
    macroaneurysm, *99, 148*
    occlusion, 66, 67, *107, 151–152*
Retinal detachment, 76–77, *105, 150*
    exudative, 76, 77
    rhegmatogenous, 76, 77
    surgical complications, *130, 162*
    tractional, 76, 77
Retinal vein occlusion, 66, 67, *103:150, 116:156*
Retinitis
    cytomegalovirus, 44, 45
Retinitis pigmentosa, 74, 75, *107, 152*
Retinoblastoma, 80, 81, *101, 149*
Retinopathy
    central serous, *134, 164*

Retinopathy (cont'd)
  diabetic, 64–65, *97*, *98*, *147*
  hypertensive, 68, 69, *142*, *167*
  of prematurity, 68, 69, *142*, *166–167*
  sickle-cell, 68, 69
Rhabdomyosarcoma, 16, 17
Rhegmatogenous retinal detachment, 76,
  77
Rheumatoid arthritis
  corneal ulceration, 36, 37
  keratoconjunctivitis sicca, 26, *112*, *154*
  scleromalacia perforans, 40, 41
Rieger's syndrome, *138*, *165*
Rodent ulcer, 8, 9
Rosacea keratitis, 36, 37
Roth spots, *129*, *161*
Rubeosis iridis, 56, 57, *116*, *155–156*

S

Salzmann's nodular degeneration, *143*, *167*
Sarcoidosis, 46, 47
Schirmer's test, 26
Sclera, blue, *131*, *163*
Scleritis, 40, 41
Scleromalacia perforans, 40, 41
Seasonal allergic conjunctivitis, 20
Sebaceous gland carcinoma, 8, 9
Seborrhoeic keratosis, 6, 7
Serpiginous choroidopathy, 48, 49
Siegrist streaks, *167*
Silicone explant, retinal surgery, *130*, *162*
Sixth nerve palsy, 88, 89
Sjögren's syndrome, 26, *112*, *154*
Solar (actinic) keratosis, 8, 9
Spring catarrh, 22, 23
Squamous cell carcinoma, 8, 9
Squamous papilloma, 6, 7
Squint *see* Strabismus, childhood
Staphylococcal infections
  blepharitis, 2, *140*, *166*
  keratitis, 28, 29
Stargardt's disease, 74, 75
Stevens–Johnson syndrome, 26, 27
Strabismus, childhood
  amblyopia, 86, *135*, *164*
  Brown's syndrome, 86, 87, *112:154*,
    118:157
  Duane's syndrome, 86, 87, *124*, *160*
  esotropia, 86, 87, *104*, *150*
  exotropia, 86, 87, *134*, *164*
Strawberry naevus, 6, 7, *117*, *156*
Stromal necrotic keratitis, 30, 31

Sturge–Weber syndrome, 58, 59
Stye, 4, 5
Subcapsular cataract, 60, 61, *103*, *150*
Subconjunctival haemorrhage, *133*,
  163–164
Superior oblique palsy, 88, 89
Suppurative keratitis, 28–29, *114*, *155*
Symblepharon, 26, 27, *153*
Syphilis, congenital, *108*, *152*

T

Terrien's marginal degeneration, *136*,
  164–165
Thiel–Behnke dystrophy, 34, 35, *124*,
  159–160
Third nerve palsy, 88, 89, *122*, *158–159*
Thyroid eye disease, 14–15, *110*, *153*
Toxocariasis, 44, 45
Toxoplasmosis, 44, 45, *129*, *162*
Trabeculectomy, 50, 51, 58, *93*, *145*
Trachoma, *143*, *167*
Tractional retinal detachment, 76, 77
Trauma
  blunt, 90, 91, *121*, *158*
  corneal abrasion, 90, 91, *122*, *158*
  foreign body, 90, 91
  orbital floor fracture, 18, 19, *100*, *148*
  penetrating, 90, *140*, *166*
Trichiasis, 12, 13
Tuberous sclerosis, 80, *98*, *148*
Tumours
  conjunctiva, 24–25, *96:146*,
    118:156–157
  eyelid, 6–9, *92:145*, *117:156*
  optic nerve head, 80, 81
  orbit, 16–17, *137*, *165*
  retina *see* Retina
  uvea, 78–79, *98*, *147–148*

U

Ultrasonography, *137*, *165*
Uveal effusion, 40, 41
Uveal tumours, 78–79, *98*, *147–148*
Uveitis
  anterior, 42–43, *114:155*, *127:161*,
    131:163
  intermediate, 46, 47
  posterior
    infectious, 44–45, *129*, *162*
    non-infectious, 46

V

Varicella *see* Herpes zoster ophthalmicus
Varices, orbital, 16, 17
Vernal keratoconjunctivitis, 22, 23
Viral wart, eyelid, 6, 7
Vitamin and mineral supplements, 70, *128,
    161*
Vitrectomy, 68, 76, *104:150, 123:159*
Vitritis, 46, 47
Vitreous haemorrhage, *123, 159*
Vitreous 'loss', *130, 162*

Vogt striae, 38, 39
Von Hippel–Lindau syndrome, 80, *94, 145*
Vortex keratopathy, *136, 164*

W

White dot syndromes, 48–49, *99:148,
    109:153*
Wilms' tumour, 58, *92, 145*
Wilson's disease, *135, 164*
Wyburn-Mason syndrome, 80